PALEONUTRITION

Method and Theory
in Prehistoric Foodways

PALEONUTRITION

Method and Theory
in Prehistoric Foodways

ELIZABETH S. WING

Florida State Museum
University of Florida
Gainesville, Florida

ANTOINETTE B. BROWN

San Pedro, California

ACADEMIC PRESS

A Subsidiary of Harcourt Brace Jovanovich, Publishers

New York   London   Toronto   Sydney   San Francisco

ACADEMIC PRESS, INC.
111 Fifth Avenue, New York, New York 10003

United Kingdom Edition published by
ACADEMIC PRESS, INC. (LONDON) LTD.
24/28 Oval Road, London NW1 7DX

Library of Congress Cataloging in Publication Data

Wing, Elizabeth S.
    Paleonutrition: Method and Theory in Prehistoric
Foodways.

    (Studies in archaeology)
    Bibliography: p.
    Includes index.
    1. Man, Prehistoric--Food. 2. Archaeology--
Methodology. 3. Indians--Food. I. Brown, Antoinette
B. , joint author. II. Title.
GN407.W56   641.3   79-21034
ISBN 0-12-759350-0

PRINTED IN THE UNITED STATES OF AMERICA

79 80 81 82   9 8 7 6 5 4 3 2 1

To Barbara Lawrence and John R. K. Robson
in gratitude for their inspiration

Contents

4 Filling Dietary Requirements

5 Human Skeletal Remains

6 Archeological Remains Related to Subsistence

7 Biological Material Used for Food

8 Procurement Patterns and Dietary Regimes

Appendix Legal Considerations Relating to the Collection, Possession, and Transportation of Biological and Archeological Specimens

Preface

Food is a concern of everyone—whether it is to stretch the food dollar, to emulate Julia Child, or to seek ways to alleviate hunger. This book has grown out of an interest in knowing how people have fed themselves in the past. To discover how people coped requires piecing together many diverse and fragmentary clues. Recognition of these clues is dependent on a combination of different research techniques and the input of specialists in various fields.

In order to bring together some of these diverse approaches to paleonutrition, we organized a symposium at the 41st Annual Meeting of the Society for American Archeology held in St. Louis, May 6–8, 1976. The symposium was entitled "Paleonutrition: The Reconstruction of Diet from Archeological Evidence." In addition to the authors in this volume, papers were presented by Joanne Bowen, Vaughn M. Bryant, Jr., Greg C. Burtchard, Dorothy J. Cattle, Stephen L. Cumbaa, Gary F. Fry, Robert I. Gilbert, Michael Kliks, Thomas Mulinski, Norman J. Sauer, Bruce D. Smith, and C. Earle Smith, Jr.

The symposium gave us the impetus and stimulation for the preparation of this book. Our objective was to cover at least briefly the types of data that have a bearing on the reconstruction of prehistoric diets. The chapters on nutrition and the evidence of nutritional status on the human body or population (Chapters 3, 4, and 5) were prepared by Antoinette Brown. The chapters concerned with the identification and analysis of archeological materials related to subsistence (Chapters 1, 2, 6, and 7) were prepared by Elizabeth Wing. The concluding Chapter 8 was a cooperative effort. Many people have contributed ideas and information that are incorporated in this book. We are most grateful to these friends and colleagues, but we alone take responsibility for what is presented in the following pages.

Acknowledgments

This book could not have been written without the encouragement of family, friends, and colleagues who have freely shared information and ideas and provided moral support for this endeavor.

Special thanks are due to a number of former University of Florida students, Stephen Cumbaa, Rochelle Marrinan, Kathleen Byrd, and Elizabeth Reitz, and Florida State Museum Technician, Sylvia Scudder, all of whom gathered data and developed methods used in probing into problems of prehistoric subsistence as well as being sounding boards for new ideas.

A number of colleagues have been kind enough to read certain chapters of this book and have provided valuable suggestions for ways in which to improve our manuscript. Jane Wheeler, Peabody Foundation, and Paul Parmalee, University of Tennessee, shared their insight, particularly into the study of biological remains from archeological sites as a source of information about subsistence. C. Earle Smith, University of Alabama, Vaughn Bryant, Texas A and M University, Edward Deevey, University of Florida, and Margaret Scarry, University of Michigan, reviewed the section on plant remains and were most generous in their help and suggestions. William Maples, University of Florida, and Cheryl Ritenbaugh, Michigan State University, provided useful comments on the section about human nutrition and osteological remains. Leslie Leiberman and Maxine Margolis, University of Florida, were most generous with their advice, particularly on human nutrition and cultural adaptations.

Thanks are also due to John F. Anderson, University of Florida, and Robert A. Martin, Fairleigh Dickinson University, for their help in determining animal biomass by scaling methods.

Legal intricacies relating to collections were most graciously explained by Michael Gordon, University of Florida Law School, and Howard Campbell, United States Fish and Wildlife Service.

Pamela Johnson, Sylvie Sidaway, and Rhoda Rybak handled all of the typing. The pains they took in getting the job done well is greatly appreciated.

We were fortunate indeed to have the artistic talents of Lynn C. Balck, who did all of the original artwork with the exception of the graphs; the graphs were prepared by Sylvia Scudder and Nancy Halliday.

Introduction **1**

As the study of human prehistory is increasingly concerned with gaining an understanding of the mode of existence of a people, greater attention is given to the most basic aspect of this, prehistoric subsistence. The subsistence system is a complex interaction between cultural concepts of what organisms are edible, technological repertoire of food procurement and preparation, and the potentials of the environment. Investigations of prehistoric foodways, while providing a more complete reconstruction of a prehistoric way of life and a time perspective to present-day problems of feeding the ever-increasing world population, require an interdisciplinary research approach, combining techniques and theories of various branches of biological, physical, and social science.

One intent of this book is to describe some of the diverse research techniques that may provide insight into prehistoric foodways. In so doing, a truly integrated approach is advocated, where the data derived from study of human, plant, and animal remains are combined with cultural data to develop a coordinated reconstruction rather than isolated and unrelated information. The importance of nonartifactual remains, such as bones, teeth, shells, and other plant and animal remains, has become widely recognized and new techniques for their analysis developed, especially during the past 2 decades since their importance was first articulated (Taylor 1957). The implications of such studies to the interpretations of prehistoric subsistence have been discussed in a number of books using primarily European data (Brothwell and Higgs 1963; Chaplin 1971; Clason 1975; Higgs 1972,

1

1975). Further indication of increased concern with such materials is evident from the greatly increased numbers of studies of this nature that are appearing in anthropological journals, and the establishment of the *Journal of Archaeological Science* in 1974 and *Human Ecology—An Interdisciplinary Journal* in 1973, which are outlets for studies relevant to human subsistence. Therefore, now is a good time to take stock of the various new interpretive techniques that have been developed and the data on which they are based. These research techniques will be illustrated primarily by examples drawn from New World prehistory prior to its discovery by Columbus.

BIOLOGICAL REQUIREMENTS FOR GROWTH AND DEVELOPMENT

The human animal is a broad-spectrum omnivore. As do all organisms, the human species has certain basic nutritional requirements, which are met in many combinations of widely varying foods, both plant and animal in origin.

A diet that will maintain a healthy condition includes 45 essential nutrients (Sebrell and Haggerty 1967) that fall into 5 different categories: (*a*) 9 amino acids in appropriate proportions and a source of nonspecific nitrogen; (*b*) carbohydrates, which are converted to the simple sugar glucose; (*c*) fats, including triglycerides and linoleic acid; (*d*) 17 minerals; and (*e*) 13 vitamins, are believed essential.

These nutrients are carried through the body in a water solution and are metabolized with oxygen to build living tissue and to provide energy. The energy required for all life processes and activities is measured in calories. The average number of calories required each day by an adult person is 2400 (ranging from approximately 1700 to 3000 calories) and depends on the individual's state of health, stage of growth and development, sex, and degree of activity. At low levels of food intake the person may function but not develop to the full genetic potential possible. Excess consumption of food is stored as fat in adipose tissue for use during lean times. Such flexibility is clearly an adaptive advantage.

AVAILABILITY OF FOOD RESOURCES

Of enormous adaptive advantage is the almost ubiquitous distribution of food sources that provide the essential nutrients for human life. Physiologically people are not bound to a single source of food, such as sloths are to cecropia leaves or a parasite to a single host. As a result, different food combinations have become established staples in various parts of the world. In Middle America, for example, the combination of corn, beans, chili peppers, and squash, supplemented by small quantities of meat or fish, has provided a well-balanced diet for many centuries. Equally nourishing is the lowland South American staple manioc (casava) supplemented by fish, or the prehistoric Andean diet based on potatoes, quinoa, and llama or guinea pig meat.

These proven diets may be adhered to for many centuries. For example, the modern Mexican diet, particularly in the rural areas, is still based on a combination of corn, beans, chili peppers, and squash despite 500 years of European influence and the introduction of new foods. When it has been possible to document dietary change in prehistoric time, change has also appeared to be gradual. Although dietary change may generally be slow, adaptability to use of new resources has made it possible for human beings to populate virtually the entire land surface of the world.

The composition of diets can vary a great deal, provided it includes the basic essential nutrients and sufficient calories. One important way in which diets differ is in respect to the proportion of meat to plant foods (Lee and De Vore 1968:43). Generally meat constitutes a very small portion of the total diet; however, important exceptions exist. The most well known are the diets of people living in extreme northern and southern temperate zones (latitudes S or N of 50°), where vegetation is sparse or totally absent and where, by necessity, the diet is composed largely of animal meat and fat. Eskimos are physiologically adapted to such a high meat diet and find a diet less high in meat difficult to tolerate. Similarly, people accustomed to a diet with little meat have difficulty changing to one composed almost exclusively of meat (Draper 1977; Nelson 1969:158). This same type of experience was described by Darwin (1962) in *The Voyage of the Beagle* during his stay with the Gauchos of Argentina.

> We were here able to buy some biscuit. I had now been several days without tasting any thing besides meat: I did not at all dislike this new regimen; but I felt as if it would only have agreed with me with hard exercise. I have heard that patients in England, when desired to confine themselves exclusively to an animal diet, even with the hope of life before their eyes, have hardly been able to endure it. Yet the Gaucho in the Pampas, for months together, touches nothing but beef. But they eat, I observe, a very large proportion of fat, which is of a less animalized nature; and they particularly dislike dry meat, such as that of the Agouti. Dr. Richardson, also, has remarked, "that when people have fed for a long time solely upon lean animal food, the desire for fat becomes so insatiable, that they can consume a large quantity of unmixed and even oily fat without nausea": this appears to me a curious physiological fact. It is, perhaps, from their meat regimen that the Gauchos, like other carnivorous animals, can abstain long from food. I was told that at Tandeel, some troops voluntarily pursued a party of Indians for three days, without eating or drinking [pp. 117–118].

Although adapting to changes in the relative amounts of meat in the diet are apparently the most difficult, other dietary changes can also be difficult, as anyone who has traveled to a different cultural area with different dietary patterns may attest. These difficulties are not only in developing antibodies to pathogens of the region, but also include adjustment of the enzyme-substrate system and bacterial flora to the types of food and their proportion in the diet. It is such experiences that make the slow evolution of diets understandable.

DEVELOPMENT OF SUBSISTENCE TECHNOLOGY AND STRATEGIES

The development of strategies and techniques for obtaining, distributing, and preparing foods is born out of a detailed familiarity with the environment. The knowledge of seasonal change in temperature and rainfall and how these affect the abundances and life histories of potential food organisms is vital to the scheduling or seasonal round of subsistence activities (Flannery 1968). People depending on the migration of caribou herds or the ascent of salmon upstream clearly must coordinate their other activities with the movements of these animals, if these animals are to play an important role in their subsistence. In less dramatic ways, perhaps, all plants and animals will be either more readily available or more useful for food during certain parts of the year. The procurement pattern must be adapted to combinations of such cycles. This adaptation can be achieved by sedentary, migratory, or transhumant ways of life.

Early agriculturalists, subsistence farmers, and pastoralists also are clearly constrained by seasonal cycles of planting, harvesting, moving animals to new pasturage, stock breeding, and innumerable other types of care that must be scheduled for successful agricultural production. Knowledge of environmental and biological seasonal changes and minor deviations from normal patterns is gained empirically. These strategies are based on knowledge of where and when resources are found. Equally important in the procurement system are the many different techniques used to obtain resources and make them available as food. The development of subsistence techniques is based on knowledge of how a resource may be obtained, nurtured, or prepared. Advances in technology may be modifications that make a simple tool vastly more effective, or innovations that make it possible to provide food for a great many more people. For example, spears are a simple type of tool that become more effective when propelled by a spear thrower or bow. Developments in technology also make available food resources that were not previously usable, for example, the development of techniques for removing the cyanide-forming agent from bitter manioc.

Innovations that have increased the food potential or reliability are irrigation systems and methods of food storage. Food storage can, of course, be viewed not only as granaries for dried grain and vats for fermented liquids but also as domestic animals and, therefore, wealth and meat stored, so to speak, on the hoof. Such innovations are associated with increased human population. Whether major innovations preceded or followed rapid population growth is debatable (Sauer 1952; Cohan 1977).

CULTURAL ATTITUDES

Cultural attitudes toward food and edible organisms and traditions that relate to every aspect of obtaining, preparing, and eating food are a part of every known social group. Many of these customs, such as religious rites and magic that help people cope with the vagaries of nature, have no tangible manifestations and will, therefore, not be possible to trace into the prehistoric past. It is, however, as important to realize the limitations to a full reconstruction of prehistoric foodways as it is to know the potential ways for interpretation of past nutrition.

RECONSTRUCTION OF PREHISTORIC DIET

> Archaeological study of Pleistocene diet is a little like navigating in the vicinity of an iceberg: more than four-fifths of what is of interest is not visible [Isaac 1971:280].

The data upon which the reconstruction of prehistoric diet are based are the identified remains of animals, plants, humans, and artifacts related to food use that are associated with a prehistoric occupation. Those remnants that provide clues about prehistoric diet are the durable, inedible portions of food, such as shell, bone, and tooth fragments of animals or grains, cobs, seeds, hulls, and rinds of plants (see Chapter 7). Characteristics of human remains that include demographic patterns, as well as skeletal and dental formation and composition, may provide clues about the nutritional status of the population (see Chapter 5). Implements for food procurement, preparation, or cooking that are associated with specific foods may be interpreted with caution as evidence for the use of the associated foods (see Chapter 6).

PRESERVATION

In the best of circumstances, these remnants are a small and disproportionate reflection of the prehistoric subsistence. All foods do not have potentially preservable inedible portions, such as bones, shell, and seeds. Some foods may be eaten or prepared and the preservable portions discarded away from the site of occupation. The process of food preparation, for example, extraction of marrow from the bone or nut from the shell, may fragment the remains, making identification difficult. Thus, at the outset the remains of past meals are unequally deposited in an occupation site.

After deposition of the discarded remains related to diet, a number of destructive forces can interfere with their recovery and study. Among these forces are mechanical destruction, such as might occur from domestic dogs scavenging scraps, traffic across the garbage deposit, and redeposition of the material as the occupation of the site changes.

After the site is abandoned, the chemical properties of the soil can influence the preservation of food remains. The acids in an acidic soil would, in time, dissolve calcium, the predominant constituent of bone. Recent work of Gordon and Buikstra (1979) has shown a direct correlation between soil pH and bone preservation in mortuary sites. In slightly alkaline soil, with a pH of 7.5, one might expect adult bone to be fragile but that most measurements of the skeletal elements will still be possible to take. The bones of young children do not fare as well. In slightly acidic soils, with a pH of 6.5, adult skeletal remains may be difficult to sex and age, while the bone of infants may be reduced to powder. Account must be taken of this differential destruction in demographic studies. Although these correlations made by Gordon and Buikstra are on human bone, a similar result may be anticipated in the effect of pH on the degree of preservation of other animal bone. The bone of young individuals is always more fragile than that of adults and therefore more subject to destruction. Likewise, all parts of a skeleton and the skeletons of all species are not equally dense and therefore unequal preservation may be expected.

The physical changes of repeated wetting–drying and freezing–thawing will also ravage bone and seed. Bone and perishable plant material are best preserved in a dry cave environment, in desert conditions, or in an anaerobic bog situation.

A number of other destructive forces bias the survival of organic material differentially. Dogs may only gnaw and thereby destroy the less dense cancellous ends of a deer femur, whereas they might completely consume a young chicken bone (Binford and Bertram 1977). Scavengers will also disperse portions of the food refuse (Isaac 1971). Trampling by the site's occupants may bury the smaller bone fragments (Gifford and Behrensmeyer 1977). Floods and erosional forces will also move different sized particles at different rates disturbing their initial orientation. As already mentioned, most bone may be dissolved in acidic soil, whereas the density of enamel will protect teeth from a similar fate. Thus, the characteristics of the organic material will be unequally affected by destructive forces.

Organic materials in archeological context are not only subject to these varied forms of destruction, but may also include biological remains not directly associated with human activity. Seeds or roots from vegetation growing near the site may be incorporated. Moles, rodents, lizards, toads, and land snails may burrow into the midden debris and perish among the cultural remains. During occupation of the site, pollen from flowering plants may be blown across the site and deposited there. Such pollen, useful in providing clues about the vegetation of the area around the site, may only indirectly indicate human use of plants.

RECOVERY

A final source of bias can result from the methods used in recovering the archeological sample. Recovery methods range in sophistication from gathering what is immediately visible and recognizable to sieving through progressively finer screen and froth flotation (Flannery 1976; Jarman, Legge, and Charles 1972). Experiments comparing the efficiency of recovering artifacts and bone by these methods clearly demonstrate an increase in the amount of cultural material recovered with the use of the finer gauge sieves (Clason and Prummel 1977; Payne 1972). The experiments described by Payne (1972) clearly showed that certain skeletal elements of large mammals (cow, pig, and sheep and/or goat) were consistently overlooked in collections picked out of the excavation trench but were recovered by sieving through a 3-mm screen. Another experiment that compared the recovery of animal bone sieved through quarter-in. screen (approximately 5 mm) and window screen (approximately 1.5 mm) followed by a flotation process resulted in a great difference in the numbers of species that were represented (Cumbaa 1973). In this study, 34 vertebrate taxa were identified. Only 8 of these were recovered using the quarter-in. mesh screen. The remaining 26 taxa would not have been represented in the faunal sample if the material had not been sieved with fine screen and the flotation process used.

These experiments demonstrate convincingly that the data base for prehistoric nutritional studies is greatly expanded by use of methods, such as sieving with fine screen, that increase the recovery of nonartifactual remains. In the study of any samples, one must be aware of the biases that may have been introduced by the recovery methods that were employed.

IDENTIFICATION

Identification of artifactual and organic material related to subsistence has intrinsic difficulties in the ease with which all the remains are recognized. Care must be taken in identifying artifacts and attributing functions to them that associate them with particular subsistence activities. Identifying pointed bone artifacts such as awls implies that they are used for piercing a material such as leather. However, such artifacts may in fact be fishing implements. On the other hand a grinding stone may typically be used for grinding corn but could also be used for grinding other grains or nuts. Prehistoric use of seines cannot necessarily be eliminated from consideration in the absence of grooved or pierced net weights. In summary, caution must be used in attributing specific functions to artifacts.

Slightly different problems must be faced in identifying biological material. Although the use to which a plant or animal was put is a matter of conjecture, a major cause of unequal treatment of biological material is the great differences in the preservation of organisms and thus the ease with which their remains can be identified. Each individual gar fish (*Lepisosteus* spp.) could contribute literally hundreds of bones and scales that can be identified to the generic level. On the other hand, there is rarely anything left of a potato. Within one broad taxonomic group, such as the bony fishes, genera exist that have many preservable and diagnostic bones in their skeletons, as in the example of the gar fish and other genera, such as, tarpon (*Megalops atlantica*). Others like the sturgeon (*Acipenser* spp.), however, have far fewer diagnostic elements. Similarly, some species may be distinguished easily on the basis of many diagnostic elements, whereas others are not as confidently identified. This is a biological problem resulting from the existing range in the degree of differentiation of different species and the extent to which this differentiation is reflected in the skeleton.

INTERPRETATION

The implications of these data to paleonutrition must be interpreted in the light of available evidence and an understanding of human nutritional requirements. Problems of differential preservation and recovery of biological remains present the main obstacles to reconstruction of prehistoric nutrition. In the absence of human remains it is not possible to assess the nutritional well being of the population. In the absence of preserved plant remains, a presumably important constituent of the diet is unrepresented. With these potentially large gaps in the data base, what accuracy can be achieved in the reconstruction of a prehistoric diet? Many details will always elude us in our attempts to fully understand a prehistoric foodway. At the same time, a number of different approaches applied to the archeological data can provide insight into a number of aspects of paleonutrition.

This interdisciplinary approach is the most productive. When remains of corn grains or cobs are absent, the evidence for use of corn may be demonstrated by the presence of grinding stones, cob-marked pottery, or radioisotope studies of human bone. Similarly, documents pertaining to an historic-period site, or written records about the community of which the site is a product, may add another dimension to the data base. Such written records, which may include plantation inventories, agricultural production figures, bills of lading of food shipments, recipes, etc., can help to corroborate and augment data derived from archeological sources. Documents relating to specific archeological sites are comparable to informants in ethnographic research in that they reflect an eye-witness account.

Use of an ethnographic model to develop an interpretation of archeological data has been criticized. The main reason for the criticism is that strict adherence to an ethnographic analogy in an archeological interpretation restricts this interpretation to known ethnographic models. In answer to such criticism Wilkinson (1975:34) argued

> that these limitations do not apply to economic prehistorians, since archaeological data represent traces of prehistoric man's participation in trophic dynamic systems, the flow of energy through which was limited by the laws of thermodynamics, with their economic and behavioral consequences for human populations. Thus, unlike students of cultural processes, the economic prehistorian has a firm basis upon which to estimate the reliability of ethnographic parallels.

Clearly one must be aware of the pitfalls in the use of ethnographic analogy. Ethnographic data can provide insight into the variety of ways people have met their subsistence needs. Ethnographic analogy may be quite valid when certain cultural adaptations are widely adhered to, and particularly when they are based on human biological characteristics. Patterns such as hunting as a male activity (Murdock 1967), food preferences and the avoidance of available and edible foods, the sharing of food, and correlation of much cultivation and consumption of maize with alkali processing techniques (Katz, Hediger, and Valleroy 1974) are all examples of subsistence patterns that have been frequently documented. Clearly this does not mean that there could never be a society in which women or children did most of the hunting, or a group which consumed everything edible that was available, or a group which did not share food, or a diet which avoids the malnutrition of maize dependence by means other than alkali treatment.

The biological requirements and energy expenditures of humans vary within relatively well-known limits. The net energy concept is therefore useful as a guide for interpretation of prehistoric subsistence (Odum 1971). The systems-ecology approach, as presented by Odum, describes and diagrams the pathways of energy flow through a natural system and the interaction between the components of the system. The theoretical basis for this approach is the laws of thermodynamics (the conservation of energy and the tendency of potential energy to degrade), Lotka's maximum power principal (the maximization of power for useful purposes as a criterion for natural selection), and general principles of ecology (community ecology and food chains). The unifying element is the energy flow that unites all interactions whether they are natural or cultural.

> In primitive agricultural systems, people spend their own energy to reduce competition between domestic plants and weeds, thereby amplifying the amount of energy trapped by the assortment of plant populations that they utilize as food. They may also supply additional nutrients when needed and where available. The interaction between energy spent by people on a given area of land and the energy available as sunlight results in the production of considerably more food than could be obtained by natural conditions. This increment in energy provided by food in turn enables people to perform even more work. In a similar manner, work spent on maintaining pasture land to raise animals for meat may also result in a net energy gain for people. Thus, in primitive agricultural communities when surpluses become repeatedly available for sale or trade, specialization may gradually develop, allowing not only for food production but also for an increasing variety of educational, political, and social activities [From Antonini, G. A., K. C. Ewel, and H. M. Tupper, *Population and energy: A systems analysis of resource utilization in the Dominican Republic,* © 1975 by University Presses of Florida, pp. 58–59.]

The network of interactions among the components of the system can be diagrammed. Such a diagram might include all the work expended in agricultural activities, such as preparing the soil, planting, weeding, eliminating competitors, harvesting, and storing the food, as well as other subsistence activities and the energy captured from all sources in the form of food. When sufficient data are available, the energy input and output can be quantified allowing computer simulation of the system. Sufficient data for quantification may rarely be available from archeological sources, but diagramming the interactions of the system is a useful way to visualize the sources and expenditures of energy.

Thus, efforts to fully understand prehistoric foodways are fraught with uncertainties. The archeological data on which such studies are based are fragmentary. This results in part from the initial use of these resources by prehistoric people. For the most part, however, data are lost through the ravages of time or through inadequate recovery. Keeping these losses in mind, we still can discover many paths that converge on reconstruction of a prehistoric foodway. Incomplete as this may be, such reconstruction still provides insight into ways in which people have met their biological needs, and how the meeting of these needs fits into their way of life and is affected by the environmental potentials and constraints.

Cultural Attitudes to Subsistence **2**

An important ingredient in the choice of food and the way it is eaten is the cultural attitude toward each food item. Many animals with flesh that, if eaten, would sustain life are not eaten because they are not considered food. Dogs in western cultures are thought of as companions, protectors, surrogate children, and innumerable other roles, but not as food. In the Orient and precolumbian Mexico, however, dogs were raised and greatly esteemed for food (Simoons 1967).

Some prohibitions are in effect for parts of the year or for particular members of the society. Turkey, which most North Americans consider an appropriate entree for the celebration of Thanksgiving and Christmas holidays, was reserved for feasts and for the elite members of society in Mexico at the time of its conquest (Duran 1967). Such distinctions in food distribution commonly fall along age and sex lines. Among the Tapirapé of Brazil, for example, "A complex set of food taboos make the job of supplying meat for a family more difficult. Children before adolescence are allowed to eat only specific meats and women are prohibited others [Wagley 1969:274]."

The well-known German proverb, *Man ist was man isst* ('One is what one eats'), expresses the universal characteristic of diets, that they are specific to a cultural group and sometimes to the different members that compose that group. The Shoshoneans give groups living in particular regions the name of the principal food consumed. The people living in western Idaho were called the groundhog eaters, while those living along the Snake River were the salmon eaters (Steward 1974:111). Dietary customs, such as food preferences and taboos, are vigorously adhered to and are generally slow to change.

When changes in diet do occur, they are often initiated by a desire for increased status that is achieved by adopting some aspects of what is viewed as an upper-class diet. Frequently the elite diet is composed of the rarest items and, therefore, the most costly in terms of money or energy required to obtain them. This is repeatedly seen as a part of patterns of acculturation. Such changes involve both deletions of foods viewed as undesirable and adaptation of desired foods. The diet of those Tepoztecans who are striving for increased status minimizes wild edible greens and maximizes the consumption of white bread (Lewis 1960:10–11). Neither of these changes improve the nutritional quality of the diet in its early transitional phase.

Just as a diet is tenaciously adhered to, methods of farming, herding, hunting, and then food sharing and eating are dictated by equally rigid customs. The procurement of food resources, whether it is hunting, farming, or another subsistence activity, has prescribed procedures. These include division of labor for the different aspects of the subsistence activity and the magico-religious beliefs observed and practiced with each of these activities. The division of labor in the major subsistence activities follows a remarkably predictable pattern. Data taken from Murdock's (1967) *Ethnographic Atlas for New World Societies* affirm the consistency with which different subsistence activities are divided among men and women of different societies (Table 2.1). Gathering of wild plants and small land animals is primarily women's work, whereas hunting, fishing, and to a lesser extent animal husbandry are primarily men's activities. Farming is done almost as

TABLE 2.1
Division of Labor in Subsistence Activities from Ethnographic Sources[a]

| Activity | Male exclusive or principal participant | | Female exclusive or principal participant | | Equal participation | | Total |
	No.	%	No.	%	No.	%	No.
Gathering	6	3	191	88	21	10	218
Hunting	304	100	0	0	0	0	304
Fishing	201	93	1	tr	14	7	217
Animal husbandry	45	67	8	12	11	16	67
Farming	49	34	61	43	33	23	143

[a] Data from Murdock 1967.

much by men as by women, and often it is a task shared equally between men and women.

These subsistence activities are accompanied, with rare exception, by magico-religious ritual of some sort. These rites are attempts to ensure the safety of the hunter or fisherman and their success in bringing a good catch or harvest in the face of so many uncertainties that have grave consequences to the social groups. These rites usually have four parts: sacrifice or offerings; prescribed behavior, which includes abstinences and/or particular observances; possession of amulets or good luck charms; and the culmination of these rites in a harvest celebration. Fragments of this ritual may be seen in Western society in the blessing of a fishing fleet, planting according to the stages of the moon, carrying a rabbit's foot, using only that favorite lure in the tackle box, and of course, the national observance of Thanksgiving. More elaborate ritual, observed by the Andean farmer, is a melding of Christian and indigenous observances that accompany every aspect of farming (Gade 1975:54). Shrines are built near the crops to ward off natural disasters, and the ritual observances include burning grass and incense and burying offerings of coca leaves and maize kernels. The phases of the moon and sun determine the agricultural calendar and are closely observed (Gade 1975:75; Murra 1975:384). The harvest is recognized by thanksgiving offerings, ceremonies, and feasting. Deviation from the accepted ritual invites danger to the crop and thereby disaster to the community.

Similar misfortune is expected by a Desana hunter in the lowlands of Colombia. The rituals a hunter must follow include: "sexual abstinence and consequently a latent state of excitation; physical cleanliness produced by bathing, emetics, and dieting; ritual purity of his weapons; the use of aromatic herbs whose perfume is exciting; facial paint; the use of tobacco; special amulets; and finally, magical invocations (Reichel-Dolmatoff 1971:220)." How much does this differ from today's affluent North American hunter who on a hunting expedition enjoys the special comraderie of a group of men equipped with prized and treasured weaponry as well as specialized clothing, face paint, and scent? Some of these observances are clearly of functional value, for example: the face painting can result in a disruptive coloration that is a camouflage; cleanliness and use of fragances mask the human scent; and various other means of heightening excitement thereby increasing adrenalin, all of which may contribute to the success of the hunter.

Comparable rites are observed by the fishermen of Martinique (Price 1966). In this case, the purpose of the ritual is to avoid or counteract witchcraft wrought by other human beings, rather than preparing the hunter to bewitch his game or propitiating the god or gods in hopes of avoiding natural disasters that would affect crops. Although the roots of the dangers to successful hunting, fishing, or agriculture are perceived as different and the details of ritual to minimize these dangers differ greatly, the basic structure of these rituals are quite similar. The Martinique fishermen have a long list of prohibitions: purification baths for the fishermen and his equipment; magic charms for the boats and fishing implements; prayers; and the coordination of fishing activities with the phases of the moon.

Another characteristic of subsistence that seems to pervade all societies is the sharing of food—a universal human trait. The rules and regulations governing the way in which food is shared are usually fairly rigid. Distribution of food beyond the nuclear family satisfies a great number of social obligations, ensures the nutritional well-being of the community, and prevents food accumulation. Among the Tasbapauni Miskito of Nicaragua the philosophy on food distribution is "if have, have to give" (Nietschmann 1973:184). In the traditional Miskito society, the distribution of food gifts is a way of life. A gift of food implies also the transmission of good luck and elicits a corresponding gift. The return gift may not, however, be of the same value, and thus there are in the community individuals who supply a major share of the food. This disproportionate share is not given nor received begrudgingly. The portions of food distributed are also unequal. The largest portions are given to close kin, particularly women relatives, and smaller shares to neighbors and godparents who are lower on the priority scale. The details of the food distribution system presented are characteristic of the traditional Miskito society and are also basically similar to food distribution among many other aboriginal groups (Nietschmann 1973). In some groups, food exchange is more strictly reciprocal, at least the exchange outside of kinship ties is (Reichel-Dolmatoff 1971:236). The giving and receiving of food may take on symbolic meaning well beyond the Miskito association of food with good luck. Among the Desana, smoked meat is symbolic of men, and smoked fish is symbolic of women. "The exchange of foods is coordinated with the rules of exchange of women; the phratries that give women must bring fish and in exchange, receive smoked meat," a symbol of the male character (Reichel-Dolmatoff 1971:236).

Symbolism associated with food pervades Western thought. The taking of bread and wine at communion, designs of sheaves of wheat on coins, "bread" as a slang term for money, Easter eggs, and decoration with ears of corn or braided wheat straws are but a few examples that will be familiar to the Western reader. Symbolism of food is likewise pervasive in most other social groups. In an Aztec ritual comparable to the Christian partaking of communion, a dough image of the great god Huitzilopochtli in the guise of a man was broken and the pieces eaten by his worshippers during the festival of the winter solstice (Frazer 1959:455).

It is a widely held belief that by consuming something it becomes a part of one. It is of course true that the nutrients in the food eaten are incorporated in the body. By extension, other characteristics associated with a prey, such as its swiftness, agility, wisdom, or courage, are commonly thought to be qualities that can be absorbed by consuming the flesh of animals that possess those traits. Foods also may be considered endowed with broader characteristics. The Desana, for example, divide their foods into male and female categories that dictate the ways in which and by whom these foods may be eaten. In similar fashion, Latin Americans under Spanish influence divide their foods into hot and cold categories that are unrelated to temperature, but that also influence the ways in which the food may be used.

The procedures observed in the butchering of animals are likewise governed by custom. In some places the job of butchering is reserved for one social class or caste, as in the Eta of Japan. In many aboriginal groups, butchering is done by the hunter or herder. Often women butcher small game, and the butchering of large game is left to the men. The sequence in the butchering procedure is usually quite standardized.

As they are practiced within a cultural group, the techniques of slaughtering domestic animals are usually uniform for each animal, but such techniques may differ between cultural groups. The Quechua-speaking Indians of Peru give the coup de grâce to their native herd animals, the llama and alpaca, by cutting across the back of the neck through the spinal cord. An atlas vertebra from the Kotosh site, dating from approximately the time of Christ, shows cut marks on its dorsal side, which may be interpreted as evidence of the antiquity of this method of slaughtering (Figure 2.1). The Eurasian methods of killing most herd animals is by slitting their throats. This method is adopted by Andean Indians when killing introduced domes-

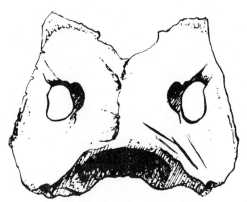

Figure 2-1. Dorsal view of a camelid atlas showing butchering scars that are evidence of the prehistoric way of slaughtering these animals at the Kotosh site in the highlands of Peru at about the time of Christ. (drawn by Lynn C. Balck)

tic animals, such as sheep and goats (Kent V. Flannery, personal communication).

The morphological difference in the llama cervical vertebrae provides a functional explanation for the traditional Andean method of slaughter. In the family Camelidae, to which llamas and alpacas belong, the neural spines of the cervical vertebrae are very low. They are so low in the axis, or second cervical vertebra, that a large gap exists on the dorsal side between the atlas, or first vertebra, and the axis, leaving the nerve cord unprotected. The Andean method of slaughter takes advantage of this anatomical feature. In other artiodactyls, such as deer and the Eurasian domesticated forms, sheep and goats, the nerve cord is protected by the large neural spine of the axis, making the severance of the nerve cord a much more difficult proposition. Thus we see that the Eurasian domesticates, sheep and goats, are slaughtered in a different manner for a particular reason, not simply tradition. Llamas could also be slaughtered by throat-slitting, but traditional methods are followed.

No less rigidly traditional is the manner in which food is prepared and eaten. Such aspects of consumption as the manner in which the food is cooked and the condiments that are used, the order in which the members of a group are served and their seating arrangement, what kinds of utensils are used, how they are held, and what kinds of thanksgiving rituals are observed are rarely haphazard. In fact, these customs are so well established that they may indicate the cultural origin, religious persuasion, and social position of a particular group within the community and of the individuals within the group.

It is clear that foods are not thought of as nutrients alone. As food is recognized as vital to existence, all activities related to food, such as procurement, preparation, and consumption, are imbued with great importance. So that the supply of food is not jeopardized, traditions related to subsistence are usually strictly observed. This may help to explain the cultural resistance to changes in subsistence, and, in turn, the discovery that subsistence is a most dependable characteristic by which to classify cultural regions and areas (Lomax and Arensberg 1977).

Nutrient Requirements 3

Humans, like other animals, have two major dietary requirements for nutrients: to supply both energy and the protein and mineral components of the body. Optimal nutrition depends on supplying essential nutrients in the correct amount and proportion when needed by the body. The proper amounts and proportions are determined by many genetic, physiological, behavioral, and environmental factors (Robson 1972).

The absolute requirement of the body for a particular nutrient may depend on the individual's weight, age, physiology, activity level, and health, and may be impossible to determine with any accuracy. As one of the factors fluctuates, for example, as activity levels rise and fall, so will the absolute requirement for a specific nutrient.

The absolute requirement can be modified by existing conditions which will necessitate additional nutrient intake. This increased requirement is known as a conditioned requirement. Increased dietary fat, for example, will impose a higher conditioned requirement for vitamin E. The absolute requirement remains the same but the conditioned requirement is greater.

Anthropologists generally refer to nutrient requirements in one of two forms: Minimum Daily Requirements or Recommended Dietary Allowance. The Minimum Daily Requirements (MDR) are legal standards, established by the Federal Food and Drug Administration for labeling foods and pharmaceutical dietary preparations. These standards specify the amounts of certain nutrients considered necessary for preventing deficiency diseases. The MDR are revised periodically and appear in Table 3.1.

TABLE 3.1
Minimum Daily Requirements of Specific Nutrients

Nutrients	Infants	Children ages 1–6	Children ages 6–12	Adults	Pregnancy/ Lactation
Vitamin A (USP)	1500.00	3000.00	3000.00	4000.00	
Thiamin (mg)	.25	.50	.75	1.00	
Riboflavin (mg)	.60	.90	.90	1.20	
Niacin (mg)		5.00	7.50	10.00	
Ascorbic acid (mg)	10.00	20.00	20.00	30.00	
Vitamin D (USP)	400.00	400.00	400.00	400.00	
Calcium (gm)		.75	.75	.75	1.50
Phosphorus (gm)		.75	.75	.75	1.50
Iron (mg)		7.50	10.00	10.00	15.00
Iodine (mg)		.10	.10	.10	.10

SOURCE: From Robson, J. R. K. *Malnutrition: Its causation and control*, Gordon and Breach, 1972.

The Recommended Dietary Allowance (RDA) represents a nutrient intake level thought adequate for healthy men and women of all ages living under normal conditions in the United States. Because of the difficulty of determining nutrient requirements for every individual in a population, the RDA were developed by the Food and Nutrition Board of the National Research Council by adding an increment (safety factor) to an average nutrient requirement. The Recommended Dietary Allowances for the United States are found in Table 3.2.

Outside the United States, many countries have established their own dietary standards. Dietary standards are nutrient intakes necessary for adequate nutrition expressed in terms of various age and physiological categories. Like the RDA, they have built-in safety factors which permit them to be applied to a population with dietary habits typical of a particular country and living under the same environmental conditions. Various countries have built different increments into their dietary standards.

On an international scale, the World Health Organization (WHO) of the United Nations has prepared recommended daily intakes for vitamins A and D, thiamine, riboflavin, niacin, ascorbic acid, vitamin B, folate, and iron. These recommendations which appear in Table 3.3, are analogous to the dietary standards of national governments. Naturally there are differences between national and international recommendations when estimating population nutrient requirements. The use of national standards is recommended whenever they are available, but, in their absence, the WHO standard should be consulted for those nutrients they publish.

In order to understand the range of human nutrient requirements, it is useful to examine in more detail the factors that influence human needs for energy and specific nutrients.

TABLE 3.2

Food and Nutrition Board, National Academy of Sciences—National Research Council Recommended Daily Dietary Allowances[a] (Revised 1968). (Designed for the Maintenance of Good Nutrition of Practically All Healthy People in the U.S.A.)

	Age[a] (years) from up to	Weight (kg)	Weight (lbs)	Height (cm)	Height (in.)	kcal	Protein (gm)	Vitamin A activity (IU)	Vitamin D (IU)	Ascorbic acid (mg)	Folacin[c] (mg)	Niacin (mg equiv)	Riboflavin (mg)	Thiamin (mg)	Vitamin B6 (mg)	Vitamin B12 (µg)	Calcium (g)	Iron (mg)
Infants	0–1/6	4	9	55	22	kg×120	kg×2.2[e]	1500	400	35	.05	5	.4	.2	.2	1.0	.4	6
	1/6–1/2	7	15	63	25	kg×110	kg×2.0[e]	1500	400	35	.05	7	.5	.4	.3	1.5	.5	10
	1/2–1	9	20	72	28	kg×100	kg×1.8[e]	1500	400	35	.1	8	.6	.5	.4	2.0	.6	15
Children	1–2	12	26	81	32	1100	25	2000	400	40	.1	8	.6	.6	.5	2.0	.7	15
	2–3	14	31	91	36	1250	25	2000	400	40	.2	8	.7	.6	.6	2.5	.8	15
	3–4	16	35	100	39	1400	30	2500	400	40	.2	9	.8	.7	.7	3	.8	10
	4–6	19	42	110	43	1600	30	2500	400	40	.2	11	.9	.8	.9	4	.8	10
	6–8	23	51	121	48	2000	35	3500	400	40	.2	13	1.1	1.0	1.0	4	.9	10
	8–10	28	62	131	52	2200	40	3500	400	40	.3	15	1.2	1.1	1.2	5	1.0	10
Males	10–12	35	77	140	55	2500	45	4500	400	40	.4	17	1.3	1.3	1.4	5	1.2	10
	12–14	43	95	151	59	2700	50	5000	400	45	.4	18	1.4	1.4	1.6	5	1.4	18
	14–18	59	130	170	67	3000	60	5000	400	55	.4	20	1.5	1.5	1.8	5	1.4	18
	18–22	67	147	175	69	2800	60	5000	400	60	.4	18	1.6	1.4	2.0	5	.8	10
	22–35[b]	70	154	175	69	2800	65	5000	—	60	.4	18	1.7	1.4	2.0	5	.8	10
	35–55	70	154	173	68	2600	65	5000	—	60	.4	17	1.7	1.3	2.0	5	.8	10
	55–75+	70	154	171	67	2400	65	5000	—	60	.4	14	1.7	1.2	2.0	6	.8	10
Females	10–12	35	77	142	56	2250	50	4500	400	40	.4	15	1.3	1.1	1.4	5	1.2	18
	12–14	44	97	154	61	2300	50	5000	400	45	.4	15	1.4	1.2	1.6	5	1.3	18
	14–16	52	114	157	62	2400	55	5000	400	50	.4	16	1.4	1.2	1.8	5	1.3	18
	16–18	54	119	160	63	2300	55	5000	400	50	.4	15	1.5	1.2	2.0	5	1.3	18
	18–22	58	128	163	64	2000	55	5000	400	55	.4	13	1.5	1.0	2.0	5	.8	18
	22–35	58	128	163	64	2000	55	5000	—	55	.4	13	1.5	1.0	2.0	5	.8	18
	35–55	58	128	160	63	1850	55	5000	—	55	.4	13	1.5	1.0	2.0	5	.8	18
	55–75	58	128	157	62	1700	55	5000	—	55	.4	13	1.5	1.0	2.0	6	.8	10
Pregnancy						+200	65	6000	400	60	.8	15	1.8	+.1	2.5	8	+.4	18
Lactation						+1000	75	8000	400	60	.5	20	2.0	+.5	2.5	6	+.5	18

SOURCE: From Robson, J. R. K. *Malnutrition: Its causation and control*, Gordon and Breach, 1972.

[a] The allowance levels are intended to cover individual variations among most normal persons as they live in the United States under usual environmental stresses. The recommended allowances can be attained with a variety of common foods, providing other nutrients for which human requirements have been less well defined. See text for more-detailed discussion of allowances and of nutrients not tabulated.

[b] Entries on lines for age range 22–35 years represent the reference man and woman at age 22. All other entries represent allowances for the midpoint of the specified age range.

[c] The folacin allowances refer to dietary sources as determined by *Lactobacillus casei* assay. Pure forms of folacin may be effective in doses less than ¼ of the RDA.

[d] Niacin equivalents include dietary sources of the vitamin itself plus 1 mg equivalent for each 60 mg of dietary tryptophan.

[e] Assumes protein equivalent to human milk. For proteins not 100 per cent utilized factors should be increased proportionally.

TABLE 3.3
Recommended Daily Intakes of Vitamins and Iron

Nutrient	Recommended intake per day	Comment
Vitamin A	750 μg retinol	1 I.U. of Vitamin A = .3 μg retinol
Thiamine	.40 mg per 1000 calories	
Riboflavin	.55 mg per 1000 calories	
Niacin	6.6 niacin equivalents per 1000 calories	60 mg of tryptophan = 1 mg niacin
Ascorbic acid		
Birth–12 years	20 mgs	
13 years and over	30 mg	
Pregnant women	50 mg	
Lactating women	50 mg	
Vitamin D		
Birth–6years	10 μg	2.5 μg of cholecalciferol = 100 I.U. of vitamin D
7 years and over	2.5 μg	
Pregnancy	10 μg	
Lactation	10 μg	
Vitamin B$_{12}$		
Birth–12 months	.3 μg	
1–3 years	.9 μg	
4–9 years	1.5 μg	
10 years and over	2.0 μg	
Pregnancy	3.0 μg	
Lactation	2.5 μg	
Folate		
Birth–6 months	40 μg	
7–12 months	60 μg	
1–12 years	100 μg	
13 and over	200 μg	
Pregnancy	400 μg	
Lactation	300 μg	
Iron		
Birth–4 months	.5 mg	
5–12 months	1.0 mg	
1–12 years	1.0 mg	
13–16 years (boys)	1.8 mg	
(girls)	2.4 mg	
Women	2.8 mg	
Men	.9 mg	
Pregnancy	2.8–6.6 mg	Depends on state of iron depletion

SOURCE: From Robson, J. R. K. *Malnutrition: Its causation and control*, Gordon and Breach, 1972.

ENERGY REQUIREMENTS

The energy demands for survival are supplied from food and measured in the form of calories. Energy demands vary with the energy needed to maintain body processes, physical activity, the energy of specific dynamic action, and the energy needed to maintain body temperature.

The published caloric allowances provide the calories to meet the normal demands but do not provide the additional needs created by stress associated with injury, infection, or disease. The higher conditioned calorie requirements provide energy for tissue repair, for immune response, and for compensation of the wasting effects of fever. In adults, the measure of caloric adequacy is the maintenance of stable body weight. In children adequate caloric intake permits a normal rate of growth throughout childhood. The measure of caloric intake that meets the conditioned caloric requirement is the rapid and complete recovery from injury, infection, or disease.

BODY PROCESSES

Adult energy requirement for maintenance of body processes include energy for basal metabolism and normal tissue growth and replacement. Children have additional energy needs for growth of new tissues. The total energy expenditure during childhood, including that for growth, is summarized in Figure 3.1.

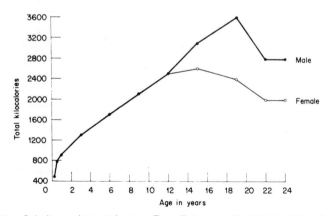

Figure 3-1. Calorie requirement by age. From Robson, J. R. K. *Malnutrition: Its causation and control,* Gordon and Breach, 1972. (Data from FAO Nutritional Studies, No. 15, 1957)

PHYSICAL ACTIVITY

Physical activity is the most variable factor in energy requirements. Energy demands for physical work may vary between one-fourth and one-half of the total energy needs.

Energy expended in physical activity is proportional to work performed. Energy requirements increase with the size of the individual, the length of time spent on the task, inefficiency of performance, and the strenuous nature of the activity. The size of the individual creates a definite variation in energy needs since more energy is required to move a larger body. Efficiency can be achieved by training and practice in the work operation, thereby reducing the necessary energy. Training may involve economizing necessary movements or reducing nonpurposeful motions, both of which may conserve energy.

Strenuous activities such as running or digging require larger amounts of energy than less strenuous ones such as writing or reading. Considerable energy may be expended in daily household tasks such as grinding grain, collecting firewood, and carrying water. In addition to this must be considered the tasks required for food production associated with farming or pastoralism. The demand for energy is seasonally variable depending on the nature of the food source. Energy requirements for various physical activities are listed in Table 3.4.

SPECIFIC DYNAMIC ACTION

After food is eaten, there is an immediate rise in heat production known as Specific Dynamic Action (SDA). One magnitude of the SDA varies with the type of nutrient and is highest for proteins. Proteins create a 30% increase in body heat. The ingestion of carbohydrates creates a 6% increase and fats 4%. The SDA of a mixture of nutrients is less than the sum of the SDA of individual constituents and is generally taken as 10% of the caloric value of food. The heat is usually wasted except in cold weather when it helps to maintain body temperature.

ENVIRONMENTAL ADAPTATION

Roughly 5% additional energy is required to perform work in ambient temperatures below about 57°F and above 99°F. In addition, there is a 2–5% increase in energy expenditure associated with carrying the extra weight and the restricting effect of cold-weather clothing and footwear.

If the body is inadequately covered, calorie needs will increase because of the increased voluntary movements to counter body cooling. At high tem-

TABLE 3.4
Energy Expenditure for Individual Activities

Operation	Calories per hour per kilogram of body weight
Work Tasks	
Sitting, writing	1.9–2.2
Typing	
manual typewriter	1.5
electric typewriter	1.3
Sweeping floors	1.7
Machine sewing	2.8
Scrubbing, kneeling	3.4
Ironing	4.2
Gardening	
weeding	4.4–5.6
digging	8.6
Ploughing with tractor	4.2
Light industry[a]	2.2–3.0
Carpentry tasks	2.2–9.1
Coal mining tasks	5.3–8.0
Transportation	
Walking	
2 mph, level surface	2.6
3.5 mph, level surface	3.6
Driving a car	2.8
Canoeing	
2.5 mph	3.0
4.0 mph	7.0
Horseback riding	
walk	3.0
trot	8.0
Cycling	
5.5 mph	4.5
9.5 mph	7.0

SOURCE: Adapted from Passmore, R. and Durnin, J. In Wohl and Goodhart (eds.), *Modern nutrition in health and disease,* Lea and Febiger, 1955.
[a] Printing, radio mechanics, shoe repair.

peratures, extra energy is expended to maintain thermal balance. Between 68–86° little adjustment is necessary.

ESTIMATING CALORIE REQUIREMENTS

Techniques used to estimate calorie requirements are based on the consumption of calories in food, or the expenditure of energy. The computation of calorie intake from the dietary intake is not feasible in paleodietary studies. Alternatively, energy expenditures are calculated from the summation of energy used in all the different types of activities. Since the direct and indirect calorimetry techniques used to determine the energy expenditure of living people cannot be applied to archeological populations, an alternative method is suggested that employs a theoretical healthy human, living in a temperate climate, as a standard (*Calorie Requirements,* F.A.O. Nutritional Study No. 15, F.A.O., Rome, 1957, Page 10).

THE REFERENCE MAN AND WOMAN

The reference man weighs 65 kg and like the reference woman, is 25 years of age and physically fit. Both live in a temperate climate having a mean annual temperature of 10°C. The reference man is in caloric balance, neither losing nor gaining weight. He works 8 hr a day but only occasionally is involved in hard labor. He is sedentary for 4 hr and spends an additional 90 min a day walking and 90 min in recreation. On the basis of this information, he is assumed to require an average of 3200 calories daily.

The reference woman weighs 55 kg and engages only in light physical

TABLE 3.5
Calorie Requirements for Subadults by Age

Age in years		Calories per day	
below 1		800	
1		900	
2		1100	
3		1300	
4		1400	
5		1500	
6		1700	
7		1800	
8		2000	
9		2100	
10		2200	
12		2500	
	Boys		*Girls*
13	2800		2600
14	3000		2600
15	3100		2600
16	3200		2500
17	3300		2500
18	3500		2400
19	3600		2400
20	3200		2200
21	3000		2100
22	2800		2100

SOURCE: Data from F.A.O. Nutritional Study No. 15, 1957.

activity, walks for 1 hour and engages in recreation for 1 hour. She requires an average of 2300 calories a day.

For infants, children, and adolescents, total caloric requirements can be expressed by age (*Calorie Requirements*, F.A.O. Nutritional Study, No. 15, 1957). The total calorie requirement increases with age until it reaches a maximum during puberty. The requirement decreases thereafter until maturity and reaches a plateau during adult life. Calorie requirements for subadults, not including the increment for physical activity, are given in Table 3.5. After the age of 12, the difference in calorie requirements for boys and girls is due primarily to larger male body size achieved during the adolescent growth spurt.

In females, the adult calorie requirement plateau may be interrupted by pregnancy and lactation. During pregnancy, extra energy is needed for the growth of the fetal and maternal tissues as well as for moving the female's additional body mass. An increased intake of 200 calories per day has been recommended for pregnant women and 600 calories daily for lactating women.

ASSESSING POPULATION REQUIREMENTS

The assessment of individual calorie requirements is liable to subjective decisions relating to activity. Attempts to assess the energy requirements of entire populations meet with more problems. The population must first be divided into groups on the basis of age, sex, physiological status, and activity levels. The respective needs for each group may then be estimated and added together. Adjustments can be made for climate and health. Inevitably, errors occur in computations of population calorie requirements, and one should, therefore, avoid a diagnosis of calorie undernutrition, or caloric adequacy based solely on a comparison of estimated caloric intake and recommended allowances for the whole population.

REQUIREMENTS FOR INDIVIDUAL NUTRIENTS

At times, a researcher may be interested in evaluating the dietary intake of a specific nutrient to test for the likelihood of under- or overnutrition. Possible nutrient deficiencies or excesses may be suggested by paleopathologies or by analogous deficiencies or excesses in contemporary populations living in the same area or practicing the same subsistence technologies.

The definition and specification of minimum requirements and dietary estimation of the requirement is almost impossible. Furthermore, the requirement may include a safety factor of known magnitude resulting in an unrealistic allowance. The intake levels of several nutrients have been decided quite arbitrarily and others are based on research that is difficult to conduct and to control. Problems of interpretation also arise because of the interrelationships of nutrients. Therefore, published nutrient-intake levels should be used as guidelines and not as tests of sufficiency.

PROTEIN REQUIREMENTS

Human protein requirements are influenced by age, body size, quality of the protein, the caloric content of the diet, and special physiological needs. Physical activity levels appear to play no special role in establishing protein needs.

The influence of age on protein requirements is especially evident in early life when protein is needed for growth of new tissues. Although the protein requirements of infants and children are high when expressed per unit of body weight, the total amount of protein is much less than that needed by an adult. Protein needs per unit of body weight decrease throughout later childhood but subsequently rise during the adolescent growth spurt. A plateau is reached in adulthood. Protein need expressed as total grams of protein is small during fetal life and infancy but increases with age until adult life. Protein requirements expressed as grams per unit body weight and as total grams are illustrated in Figures 3.2 and 3.3.

Protein needs of pregnant or lactating women are greater than those of other adult women. Sufficient protein must be eaten to provide for the

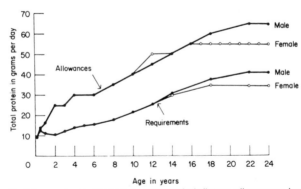

Figure 3-2. Protein requirements and recommended dietary allowances by age and sex. From Robson, J. R. K. *Malnutrition: Its causation and control,* Gordon and Breach, 1972. (Data from World Health Organization Technical Report Series, No. 301, 1965 and *Recommended dietary allowances,* Seventh Edition, National Academy of Sciences, Washington, D.C.)

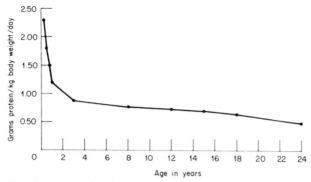

Figure 3-3. Reference protein requirements by age. From Robson, J. R. K. *Malnutrition: Its causation and control,* Gordon and Breach, 1972. (Data from World Health Organization Technical Report Series, No. 301, 1965).

mother's own needs as well as those of the growing fetus. During lactation the female must also supply the protein used in the synthesis of milk.

An increase in body size increases needs for tissue repair and normal maintenance and replacement. Since the male is generally larger, he will need more total protein. Both malnutrition and illness can cause increased protein requirements. Extra protein is used in the immune response to disease organisms, as well as for both tissue repair and replacement of tissue in a person recovering from illness.

PROTEIN QUALITY

Both the quantity and quality of dietary protein are important variables in determining the availability of protein to meet individual requirements. Protein serves as a source of amino acids for building and repairing tissues. Protein can also provide energy when other energy sources (fats and carbohydrates) are inadequate. The human body requires protein in order to provide specific amounts and proportions of the essential amino acids contained in proteins. Protein requirements, therefore, are defined by needs for essential amino acids that cannot be synthesized from the other nonessential amino acids. The essential and nonessential amino acids are listed in Table 3.6.

Protein quality is evaluated by the proportion of its component amino acids. A balanced protein such as that of milk or egg contains amino acids in the proportion required by the human body. Other food proteins may be imbalanced with respect to one or more amino acids.

Deficiencies in protein quality can only be compensated for by providing other proteins that supply the deficient amino acids. Protein of low biological value (imbalanced) is usually present in low concentrations in the diet. As a result, practical difficulties arise in consuming sufficient quantities of

TABLE 3.6
Essential and Nonessential Amino Acids

Essential	Nonessential
Valine	Glycine
Threonine	Alanine
Leucine	Serine
Isoleucine	Cysteine
Methionine	Tyrosine
Phenylalaine	Proline
Lysine	Hydroxyproline
Tryptophan	Arginine
Histidine[a]	Glutamic acid
	Aspartic acid
	Cystine

[a] Essential only for infants.

the food to meet the needs for the limiting amino acids (those amino acids present in the lowest concentration).

INTERRELATIONSHIPS OF NUTRIENTS

Nutritional requirements are influenced not only by growth and extraneous factors such as disease and climate, but also by the presence, concentration, and function of other nutrients.

Interrelationships between energy intake, protein intake, and several vitamins have been observed. In addition, there are also interactions between vitamins and energy requirements that affect the respective requirements for these nutrients.

VITAMINS AND MINERALS

The roles of thiamine, riboflavin, and niacin in energy metabolism imply that requirements of these vitamins are related to human energy needs and expenditures. Not only is the requirement for thiamine related to the total caloric intake but also to the proportions of fat, carbohydrate, and protein in the diet. As the carbohydrate portion of the diet increases, more thiamine is required for its metabolism. Conversely, thiamine requirements are reduced whenever other sources of calories are substituted for carbohydrates.

The total caloric requirement is related to body weight and activity levels, and the thiamine requirement varies accordingly. The increased energy expenditure associated with pregnancy increases the need for thiamine, as does lactation.

Niacin requirements are not only related to energy and protein intake but also to amino acid intake. The amino acid tryptophan can be converted by the body to niacin in the absence of dietary niacin.

Pyridoxine (vitamin B_6) is also involved in protein metabolism. The requirement for this vitamin is related to total protein intake and increases from infancy through childhood into adulthood and again with pregnancy and lactation. The presence of infections which initiate an antibody response creates extra demands for protein and therefore pyridoxine.

The requirement for vitamin A is related to several other nutrients. The level of dietary fat is important since it facilitates the intestinal absorption of carotenes which are precursors of vitamin A available from plant sources. There are also direct relationships between the level of protein intake and the need for vitamin A. An ample allowance for protein will promote rapid growth in childhood, which demands extra vitamin A. On the other hand, very low protein intake can result in poor vitamin A utilization since protein is necessary for vitamin A absorption, mobilization in the liver, and its transport within the body.

Vitamin C (ascorbic acid) facilitates the absorption of some of the iron in vegetables. Communities depending on vegetables as their source of iron may have a higher vitamin C requirement than those whose iron is contained in animal sources.

Vitamin D facilitates the absorption of calcium and phosphorus from the small intestine and aids in the normal deposition of these minerals in bones and teeth. Increased consumption and need for these minerals, especially in pregnancy and lactation, and during growth, increases the need for vitamin D to aid in their utilization.

The efficient use of calcium and phosphorus depends on the ratio of one mineral to the other. A calcium intake roughly equal to the intake of phosphorus is considered optimal for utilization of both nutrients. A predominance of phosphorus is poorly tolerated and can lead to an increase in the requirement for calcium.

Energy can be produced from proteins, fats, or carbohydrates. The body places such importance on the maintenance of energy production that even though the body will be deprived of protein for tissue growth and repair, protein will be diverted and used as a source of energy in the absence of dietary fats and carbohydrates. Protein adequacy cannot be assessed solely on the basis of quantitative measurement of protein intake. If there are not enough calories in the diet from fats and carbohydrates, the deficit in energy will be made up from protein.

BIOLOGICAL ADAPTATION TO DIETARY INTAKES

The discrepancy observed between known intakes and estimated requirements of nutrients in many populations may be due in part to physiological adaptation. The requirement for calcium as determined by experimentation is much higher than the known intakes of calcium for many communities. The ability to maintain an adequate calcium balance (intake equal to loss) can be attributed to small body size and increased efficiency of absorption and utilization, and perhaps reduced loss. In many areas where diets are poor in calcium, the skeleton is small, resulting in a lower absolute requirement for calcium. In addition, metabolic adaptation to low intakes of calcium results in greater efficiency of absorption and utilization.

Similarly, the estimated requirements for iron are influenced by the availability of iron in the food and by the ability of the body to control iron absorption. Despite low intakes of iron, an adequate status can be achieved by facilitated absorption of the element.

In nitrogen balance studies, it has been demonstrated that the body can adapt to a lowered protein intake. Although there may be a temporary period of negative nitrogen balance during which nitrogen loss exceeds protein intake, equilibrium may be restored at this lower level of intake. Balance is restored through reduced loss and increased absorption and utilization.

If the intake is reduced again, the body will once more go into negative nitrogen balance and further adaptation may take place. The ability of the body to adapt appears dependent on the levels of protein intake prior to the deprivation. Persons on high intakes go into negative nitrogen balance on a higher level of protein intake than subjects who have habitually consumed a low-protein diet.

Biological adaptation to low levels of caloric intake occurs at many levels. Acute calorie shortages cause breakdown of stored fat and eventually stored protein in the form of muscle for use in filling energy requirements. Continued calorie shortages may result in reduced activity levels which temporarily lower the individual's caloric requirements. Chronic low-calorie intakes during childhood result in small body size which reduces the absolute calorie requirement of the undersized adult.

DISTURBANCES IN METABOLISM

Failure to absorb and utilize nutrients may result from inborn errors of metabolism, or from disease states which interfere with normal metabolism.

Disturbances of metabolism generally cannot be compensated for by biological adaptation. Instead, metabolic disturbances may impose a higher conditioned requirement for a particular nutrient or may require removal of a particular food from the diet. If no compensation or correction of the disturbance is possible, permanent damage may result to the individual.

CARBOHYDRATES

DIABETES

This disorder is due to a reduction in the production of insulin; consequently, less glucose enters the cells and accumulates, instead, in the bloodstream. The elevation of blood sugar level (hyperglycemia) may be so high that the kidney tubules become overloaded. Above a concentration of 180 mg per 100 ml of blood, the sugar will spill over into the urine.

Two types of diabetes are recognized. Diabetes insipidus is caused by infection, tumor, trauma, or congenital disorder that disturbs normal pituitary function and the secretion of antidiuretic hormone, resulting in the passage of large quantities of urine.

Diabetes mellitus is characterized by multiple metabolic disturbances resulting from an insufficiency in the supply of insulin secreted by beta cells of the Islets of Langerhans of the pancreas. It is rare in infancy, uncommon in childhood, and most common in adults over 50 years of age.

Most cases of diabetes mellitus are genetic in origin, but a few may be attributed to pancreatic disease or to disturbances in the endocrine function of the pituitary and adrenal glands. The predisposition to diabetes is inherited, and hyperglycemia occurs when the individual is faced with some extraneous stimuli, such as the stress of pregnancy or obesity.

Humans may originally have been able to convert to stored fat the small amounts of carbohydrate available in the pre-agricultural diet. Modern agriculture produces large amounts of carbohydrates that are frequently consumed in excess of caloric requirements, resulting in the formation of excess fatty deposits. Perhaps in former times of more temperate food consumption, people were protected from diabetes.

FRUCTOSE

Fructose contributes between one-sixth and one-third of the total carbohydrate content of most human diets. More than 50% of fructose is metabolized by a specific fructose pathway. In some persons, one of the enzymes in this pathway is deficient, so that an abnormally high level of fructose accumulates in the blood. Eventually, this may result in fructosuria, the appearance of fructose in the urine.

In fructose intolerance, a separate condition, a liver enzyme deficiency is involved which permits fructose to accumulate in the cells without being converted into glucose, creating hypoglycemia.

GALACTOSEMIA

Galactosemia is the result of a deficiency of an enzyme which converts galactose-1-phosphate to glucose-1-phosphate. Galactose-1-phosphate consequently accumulates in the blood, while at the same time, blood-glucose level is lowered. This inherited disease is noticed soon after birth, when ingested milk, the principal source of galactose, causes vomiting and diarrhea. Continued milk ingestion results in hypoglycemia which causes jaundice and liver enlargement, the formation of cataracts in the lens of the eye, and mental retardation.

GLYCOGEN-DEPOSITION DISEASE

A group of diseases is associated with the genetic absence of an enzyme, most often glucose-6-phosphatase, involved in the metabolism of stored glycogen. The absence of the enzyme leads to an excessive accumulation of glycogen in the liver and other organs and tissues.

DISACCHARIDASE DEFICIENCY

The genetic deficiency of any one of the disaccharidases (maltase, lactase, and sucrase) prevents digestion of that particular disaccharide (maltose, lactose, or sucrose). The osmotic pressure of the unabsorbed sugar retains water in the intestine, producing diarrhea. Unabsorbable sugar, broken down by bacteria in the colon into smaller molecules, causes an additional increase in osmotic pressure, and the bacteria produce organic acids and gas which lead to passage of watery and foamy stools. Other symptoms are vomiting, abdominal distention, and cramps.

Lactase deficiency occurs in both the juvenile-onset and adult-onset forms. It is generally thought that the original human condition is adult-onset lactase deficiency, as it is for the other primates. In adult-onset lactase deficiency, lactose, present in human milk, can be digested until the child reaches the age of 12 or so. After that, lactase is no longer produced in quantities sufficient to digest more than a cup or so of milk at a time. Ingestion of large quantities of milk produces the symptoms of disaccharidase deficiency. The production of lactase into adulthood is the result of a gene which arose in the past and increased in frequency in those populations which had access to large quantities of unprocessed animal milk. These were most likely herding populations who would have been able to take advantage of the calories available in animal milk to supplement or even form a large part of their diet. In populations in which adults remain lactose intolerant, either animal milk was never available in sufficient quantities for the gene to be advantageous, or milk was processed to produce yogurt or cheese, thereby breaking down the lactose before human ingestion (Cook 1978; Lisker, Gonzales, Daltabuit 1975; Neale 1968).

AMINO ACIDS

PHENYLKETONURIA

Because of a hereditary lack of the enzyme phenylalanine hydroxylase, the normal oxidation of phenylalanine to tyrosine in the liver cannot occur. Consequently, phenylalanine accumulates in the serum and excessive amounts of some of the metabolites of phenylalanine are excreted in the urine. Unless phenylalanine is eliminated from the diet, severe mental retardation may occur as phenylalanine metabolites attack the brain cells.

ALCAPTONURIA

In the absence of the enzyme homogentisic acid oxidase, homogentisic acid, metabolite of phenylalanine and tyrosine, cannot be further broken down, either in the liver or the kidney. As a result, homogentisic acid accumulates in the blood, and spills over into the urine. Cartilage and other connective tissue becomes pigmented, and the individual is susceptible to arthritis in later life.

ALBINISM

Albinism results from insufficient production of the enzyme tyrosinase, which produces the metabolites of tyrosine needed by melanocytes to produce normal quantities of the pigment melanin which colors the skin, hair, and eyes. Unlike the other amino-acid enzyme deficiencies, albinism does not result in the accumulation of tyrosine in the blood serum, since alternative pathways exist for it to be either oxidized or converted into epinephrine or thyroxine.

MAPLE-SYRUP URINE DISEASE

An inborn error of metabolism blocks the oxidative decarboxylation of branched chain amino acids (leucine, sioleucine, and valine) resulting in their accumulation, as well as that of their associated alpha-keto acids. Large amounts of this accumulation spill over into the urine, hence the name. The disease, which may be fatal, becomes apparent in infancy and survivors are mentally retarded.

HISTIDINEMIA

Due to the genetic lack of the enzyme histidase, histidine cannot be metabolized. As a result, histidine accumulates in the blood serum, and as in most amino-acid enzyme deficiencies, histidine and certain of its metabolites are excreted in the urine. Individuals who inherit this disease develop mental retardation and speech difficulties.

OTHER INHERITED DISEASES

Other more common disorders of amino-acid metabolism include prolinemia, hydroxyprolinemia, cystathionuria, homocystinuria, and deficiency of urea cycle enzymes, all of which result in mental retardation.

UNDERNUTRITION AND OVERNUTRITION

Nutrient adequacy is a balance between consumption and expenditure or loss. Chronic underconsumption or overconsumption of nutrients may result in conditions to which the body cannot adapt successfully within its range of physiological adaptations. In these cases clinical syndromes appear. The limitations of this chapter permit discussion of only the most common nutritional diseases.

ENERGY DEFICIENCY

The chronic failure to consume the calories necessary to fill energy requirements leads to protein-calorie malnutrition, perhaps the most widespread of all deficiency diseases. If caloric intake is inadequate to meet the demands of the body, any available nutrient will be broken down to create energy. A diet lacking in calories will lead to the use of stored fat and ingested protein for energy. When these sources are unavailable or exhausted, protein in the form of muscle tissue will eventually be broken down (muscle wasting) for conversion into energy.

A diet containing inadequate calories is liable to be deficient in many essential nutrients resulting in multiple nutrient deficiencies. Consequently, protein caloric malnutrition is a syndrome with many clinical manifestations.

When the main deficiency in the diet is caloric, growth stops and the affected child is usually thin and short for his or her age. Clinically, this condition is known as marasmus. If, on the other hand, caloric intake is adequate, but protein is lacking either in quantity or quality, not only does the child fail to grow, but also displays signs of disturbed body function such as edema (water retention), skin lesions, and muscle wasting beneath perhaps normal amounts of subcutaneous fat. Such a condition is known as kwashiorkor. Between these two extreme syndromes lie intermediate forms which may be complicated by other nutrient deficiencies. Caloric inadequacy of the marasmus form is more likely to affect infants whose mothers fail to lactate or who are fed inadequate amounts of breast milk substitute. Consequently, marasmus is seen mainly in infants under 1 year of age.

After about 6 months of age, breast milk is inadequate to supply all the growing child's nutrient requirements. When weaning to solid food is delayed, or when the weaning diet contains protein either low in quantity or quality, kwashiorkor develops. Because the development of kwashiorkor takes time, it is more prevalent in the second year of life, although marasmic children may also appear in this age group, just as infants and children in the first year of life may also suffer from kwashiorkor.

The mortality rate for children suffering from protein calorie malnutrition is high, not only due to death from frank starvation, but also because the malnourished child is more likely to die from childhood diseases from which normally nourished children recover. A high mortality rate from measles, for example, would not be uncommon among children suffering from some forms of protein-calorie malnutrition.

Although there may be complete recovery from protein-calorie malnutrition if calories in excess of those required are provided to permit "catch-up" growth to occur, it is more common for the malnourished child to be always shorter than normal children of the same age (Krueger 1969).

ENERGY EXCESS

When energy intake exceeds expenditure, the energy is stored as body fat and the person gains weight. The body has no mechanism for excreting excess energy as it does for excess water or minerals. The clinical condition of positive energy balance is known as obesity. Genetic influences seem to play a role in predisposition to obesity, as does geography, climate, and culture, all of which affect food intake and activity levels. Ethnicity has a bearing on the prevalence of obesity, as does socioeconomic status. Differences have also been observed between the sexes. While the influence of these factors is far from understood, it is clear that overweight infants tend to be born of heavy parents. The overweight infant tends to become an overweight child who, in turn, tends to become an overweight adolescent and adult.

The exact prevalence of obesity cannot be determined accurately as there are no standardized criteria for obesity. The immediate effects of obesity are reflected in problems of locomotion and liability to serious injuries during accidents. Obesity also produces progressive changes in pulmonary function (Wilson and Wilson 1969). In time, changes in the joints are likely to occur because of the excessive weight-bearing strains. Cardiovascular and renal diseases have been noted as being almost twice as prevalent in the obese as in the non-obese, although this is only an association and not a causal relationship.

THE VITAMINS

The distinctions between hypervitaminosis, vitamin sufficiency, and hypovitaminosis, are unclear and ambiguous. The vitamin-deficiency diseases are clinical manifestations that may develop months after negative vitamin balance first begins. During that time the individual suffers from depletion of the body stores of that vitamin, and the tissues become deficient. Between hypovitaminosis and hypervitaminosis lies a nebulous condition of vitamin sufficiency in which the individual displays no clinical signs. The actual condition, however, may range from borderline hypovitaminosis, in which the individual requires more vitamin than is being ingested, to a vitamin balance, in which the body is utilizing all the ingested vitamin, to tissue saturation, in which the tissues contain all the vitamin they can carry, to storage saturation, in which body stores are filled to maximum capacity. Continued excess consumption of the vitamin will lead to the clinical signs associated with hypervitaminosis, but again, many months may pass before the pathological condition becomes apparent. It is important for archaeologists, who see only the clinical signs impressed on the bone, to remember the gradual processes involved.

Only the more common vitamin-disease conditions will be discussed. The others are indicated in Table 3.7. Deficiencies of any of the vitamins may occur, but it is less likely that excesses of the water-soluble vitamins will occur since storage of these vitamins is more limited.

VITAMIN A

In humans, hypovitaminosis A affects the retina of the eye, the conjunctiva, and the cornea. In the early states of the disease, the efficiency of the

TABLE 3.7
Summary of Hypovitaminosis and Hypervitaminosis Syndromes

	Hypovitaminosis	Hypervitaminosis
Fat-soluble vitamins		
Vitamin A	Night-blindness, xerophthalmia, keratomalacia, bone malformation, growth retardation	Muscle and joint pains, skin changes, weight loss, liver enlargement
Vitamin D	Rickets, osteomalacia, osteoporosis	Bone demineralization, growth retardation, soft tissue mineralization
Vitamin E	Anemia	
Vitamin K	Hemorrhage	
Water-soluble vitamins		
Ascorbic acid	Scurvy	
Thiamine	Beri-beri	
Riboflavin	Cheilosis, glossitis, angular stomatitis, eye changes	
Niacin	Pellagra	
Biotin	Dermatitis, muscle pain, anemia	
Pyridoxine	Anemia, convulsions, dermatitis	
Pantothenic acid	Cramps, depression, insomnia	
Folic acid	Megaloblastic anemia	
Vitamin B$_{12}$	Pernicious anemia	

light-sensitive rod cells in the retina is impaired, resulting in night-blindness. In later stages, the conjunctiva become thickened, producing xerosis conjunctival. In severe deficiency, suffered by many infants, the xerosis does not have time to develop. Instead, the cornea dries and structural damage to the surface follows. The corneal involvement of the eye is termed xerophthalmia, and is characterized by a dry and lusterless condition of the eyeball.

Hypovitaminosis A mainly affects the poor of South and East Asia, and, to a lesser extent, urban concentrations in the Near East, Latin America, and Africa.

VITAMIN B COMPLEX

Beri-beri is usually described as two distinct clinical syndromes of thiamine deficiency, depending on whether the nervous system or the cardiovascular system is affected. The clinical syndrome affecting the nervous system is usually termed dry beri-beri, while the cardiovascular manifestations are usually referred to as wet beri-beri. Dry beri-beri is characterized by muscular weakness, painful muscles, and paralysis of the limbs, in contrast to wet beri-beri typified by edema and cardiac failure.

Infants born of thiamine-deficient mothers are liable to contract beri-beri. Because the breast milk fails to supply sufficient thiamine to meet the infant's requirements, infantile beri-beri follows. In affected infants, cardiac failure and labored breathing are often followed by death.

In the past, beri-beri was found in parts of Asia where rice was polished before consumption. Thiamine is located in the outer layers of the rice grain, which are removed during the polishing process. Consequently, polished rice is seriously deficient in thiamine. As polished rice became more widely consumed, beri-beri became a more serious public health problem except where parboiling is practiced. During parboiling, the rice is treated with heat and water, resulting in the movement of the water-soluble thiamine from the outer layers to the inner part of the grain, which is not affected by the polishing process.

Pellagra, a deficiency disease caused by inadequate nicotinic acid and tryptophan, is endemic in parts of the world where the staple diet of the poor is maize. Pellagra is characterized by loss of weight, skin lesions, and gastrointestinal and mental disturbances. In chronic cases, there may be degenerative changes in the nervous system, causing disturbances of sensation and muscle paralysis.

The exact relationship of nicotinic acid to pellagra is not perfectly understood. It has been suggested that the nicotinic acid in maize may not be available to the body. This would explain why pellagra occurs in maize eaters and not others who consume cereals containing less nicotinic acid than maize.

Megaloblastic anemia can result from a deficiency of either folic acid, which is necessary for the formation of hemoglobin, or from a deficiency of vitamin B_{12}, which controls folic-acid enzymes. Megaloblastic anemia is characterized by low hemoglobin level and the presence of large and immature red blood cells. Megaloblastic anemia, caused by vitamin B_{12} deficiency, may be complicated by severe neurological disturbances following degeneration of the spinal cord.

Megaloblastic anemia is rarely the result of either folic-acid or vitamin B_{12} deficiencies in the diet. It does occur, however, when there are extra demands for these nutrients, as during pregnancy and lactation. It may also result from malabsorption of either nutrient.

VITAMIN C

Deficiency of vitamin C (ascorbic acid) leads to the development of the clinical condition known as *scurvy*. Without sufficient vitamin C, the body is unable to maintain connective tissue, producing pathological changes. In the bones and teeth, growth and continued development is prevented by the lack of supporting connective tissue. The teeth become loose, and may be lost because the tissue that normally holds them firmly in the jaw is lacking. The supporting tissue in the walls of the smaller blood vessels and capillaries also fails. Consequently, vessels and capillaries are liable to rupture, causing blood to escape into the surrounding tissue.

Fruits, vegetables, and tubers, the principal sources of vitamin C, are generally seasonal, which often leads to seasonal deficiencies of the vitamin. Furthermore, vitamin C is unstable and soluble in water, leading to its destruction during processing and cooking. Consequently, vitamin C deficiency is more common among populations heavily dependent on processed and preserved foods. Scurvy also occurs in infants who have been fed on cow's milk alone, without supplementary sources of ascorbic acid.

VITAMIN D

The relationships between vitamin D, and the minerals calcium and phosphorus must be considered when discussing the deficiency diseases of *rickets, osteomalacia,* and *osteoporosis.* Rickets affects infants and children, whereas osteomalacia affects adults, usually pregnant and lactating women, and osteoporosis affects the elderly.

Humans obtain vitamin D either by ultraviolet radiation of sterols in the skin, or from ready-made dietary sources. If vitamin D deficiency occurs through a breakdown in either of these two sources, the absorption of calcium and phosphorus from the gut is impaired. Since vitamin D is fat-soluble, disturbance in fat absorption will also interfere with vitamin D absorption from dietary sources. The multiple deficiencies of vitamin D, calcium, and phosphorus cause disturbance in the mineralization of cartilage that normally becomes bone. In an attempt to maintain proper serum calcium levels, calcium is withdrawn from existing bone, leading to its destruction.

The clinical features of rickets may include cessation of bone growth, widening of the epiphyses of the forearm bones at the wrist, and swellings at the junction of the rib cartilages and the breast bone. The withdrawal of calcium from the skull bones results in their becoming softened, and later the skull may show protuberances of the forehead known as bossing. The development of the teeth is affected, delaying their eruption.

Continuation of the deficiency is accompanied by secondary complications. The softened limb bones are unable to support the weight of the body and they become bowed. Similarly, the rib cage may be deformed, producing a bowed "pigeon chest" which may hinder proper breathing. Thus, upper respiratory infections become an important and sometimes terminal feature of rickets. In the female child, the weight stress on the pelvic bones can cause pelvic deformities which may hinder or prevent normal parturition during adulthood.

Osteomalacia is a disease of adult life. Females, because of the extra demands for calcium and vitamin D during pregnancy and lactation, are essentially prone to the disease. The deficiency leads to a failure of the body to deposit calcium in the cartilaginous bone matrix. Pain in the feet and in the lumbar region of the spine are common. The limb bones are particularly liable to fracture. Radiological examination reveals the typical picture of generalized rarefaction and irregularities which resemble bone fractures.

Osteoporosis is a clinical syndrome, usually found in the elderly, which results from a loss of mineral from the bones. Although osteoporosis is especially prevalent in postmenopausal females, both sexes of advancing age may be affected. There is generalized rarefaction of the bones, accompanied by pain and frequent fractures. It has been shown that vitamin D may play a part in the etiology of this disease. In addition to low vitamin D intakes and inadequate irradiation, we must take into account malabsorption, inadequate dietary calcium, and inactivity.

Rickets and osteomalacia occur in populations consuming poor diets, and in regions where the opportunity for irradiation of the skin by sunlight is poor, either due to excessive cloud cover, high buildings blocking the sun, seclusion indoors, heavy clothing, or atmospheric pollution. Diets lacking milk or dairy products are associated with rickets. Cereal diets are especially dangerous to children with marginal calcium intakes since the phytates contained in cereals may interfere with calcium absorption.

MINERALS

The situation with regard to mineral sufficiency is similar to that for vitamins. A subclinical deficiency may impair normal growth and development or function, but may not leave scars on the bones to prove its presence. Similarly, hypermineralosis may produce visible clinical signs, but may not be recognized from the skeletal remains without analysis of the mineral content of the bone. Only the most common of the mineral syndromes will be presented (Table 3.8).

IRON

A deficiency of iron leads to the clinical condition of *anemia*. In iron-deficiency anemia, the red blood cells are normal in size, but they are deficient in the oxygen-carrying pigment hemoglobin.

TABLE 3.8
Summary of Hypomineralosis and Hypermineralosis Syndromes

Mineral	Hypomineralosis	Hypermineralosis
Calcium	Rickets, osteomalacia, osteoporosis, tetany	
Phosphorus	Rickets, bone fragility	
Magnesium	Vasodilation, soft tissue mineralization, atherosclerosis, tetany	
Sodium	Nausea, anorexia, muscular weakness, cramps	Hypertension
Potassium	Weakness, anorexia, abdominal distention, tachycardia	
Iron	Anemia	Nutritional cytosiderosis
Copper	Anemia, demyelination of nerves, bone disorders	
Manganese	Ataxia	
Zinc	Hepatosplenomegaly, dwarfism, hypogonadism	
Iodine	Goiter, cretinism	
Fluorine	Dental caries	Fluorosis, dental staining, dental pitting, increased bone density, soft tissue mineralization
Cobalt	Anemia	
Chromium	Impaired glucose tolerance curve	
Molybdenum	Poor growth	
Selenium	Growth retardation	

Mild anemia produces lassitude, but more severe cases show signs of inadequate cardiac function. The deficiency of iron may lead to other disturbances of function caused by a lack of enzymes that depend on iron.

Iron deficiency anemia is extremely prevalent and is a serious public health problem in most nonindustrialized and tropical regions. The exact prevalence of anemia is impossible to assess due to differing criteria and measurement techniques world-wide.

Iron-deficiency anemia affects persons of all ages and physiological states. An infant is born with an iron endowment from the mother. Low birthweight babies have smaller amounts of iron than those of normal weight and are consequently more likely to become anemic. Infants fed past the first 6 months of life on a diet of only milk will be unable to meet their iron requirements and will become increasingly anemic unless supplementary iron is added from other dietary sources.

A lack of sufficient animal protein in the diet may add to the risk of anemia, because it is believed that the presence of animal foods in the diet enhances the absorption of iron in vegetable foods. An overall protein deficiency in the diet leads to a decrease in the quantity of the protein compound transferrin which is responsible for transporting iron in the blood. A lack of transferrin may contribute to the development of iron-deficiency anemia as may the additional demands for iron imposed by growth, pregnancy, hemorrhage, and parasites.

TRACE ELEMENTS

IODINE

From a point of view of prevalence, deficiency of the trace element iodine is a serious problem. The thyroid gland responds to deprivation of iodine by cell multiplication and physical enlargement. At first, the enlargement may be diffuse and cause no disability, but as the iodine deficiency continues, the enlargement becomes visible and a large goiter may develop which can interfere with swallowing, respiration, and movement of the neck.

Goiter is more common in females, especially during adolescence and pregnancy. In areas where goiter is endemic, iodine deficiency can cause severe effects known as cretinism which is characterized by retarded physical and mental development. Cretinism usually occurs among the offspring of women who are suffering from goiter, which suggests that the damage to the child took place before birth.

Goiter is endemic in many parts of the world where geological and climatic events have deprived the soil of iodine. The principal endemic goiter regions of the world are the Alps in Europe, the Himalayas in Asia, the Andes in South America, the Rocky Mountains of North America, and the Highland areas of the Philippines and New Guinea. It is also found in the plains around the Great Lakes of North America and in other isolated localities where the water supply is hard. This condition is portrayed in the Adena figure from prehistoric Ohio (Figure 3.4). Although seafoods are good sources of iodine, the proximity of the sea does not exclude the possibility of goiter.

The development of goiter is not a simple matter of dietary iodine deficiency. In some cases, the prevalence of goiter has been attributed to hard water, in others, to the presence in the diet of substances antagonistic to the thyroid gland. The consumption of milk from animals fed on these foods may also lead to the development of goiter. These goitrogenic agents are contained in the leaves and seeds of plants of the cabbage family.

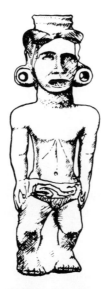

Figure 3-4. Iodine deficiency as reflected in the goiter and other physical changes is clearly portrayed in the figure from an Adena site in Ohio. (drawn by Lynn C Balck by permission of the Ohio Historical Society. The Adena figure is in the Ohio Historical Society Collection)

ZINC

Deficiency of zinc retards growth in children and retards development of the male genitals. Zinc is present in newborns' tissues, and was received from the mother, but losses of zinc in early life are not recovered from breast milk, which is poor in zinc. In the Middle East, zinc deficiency has been attributed to the predominance of vegetable foods, such as cereals and legumes, which contain zinc in an unavailable form. The malabsorption caused by the binding of the zinc to other compounds may be aggravated by the presence of excess calcium. The presence of dietary animal protein, on the other hand, enhances zinc absorption.

FLUORINE

Fluorine is normally deposited in the bones and teeth, so these are the areas affected by excessive fluorine intake. In the early stages of fluorosis, or fluoride poisoning, the teeth show opaque white flecks in the enamel. In later stages, the teeth become stained with a brown pigment. In the advanced stages, the teeth are pitted and have a corroded appearance. There is an increase in bone density and overgrowth of bone. Joints may become immobilized when the ligaments and tendons become calcified. Neurological disturbances of the spine can be caused by the bony overgrowths of the vertebrae which interfere with the nerve trunks as they leave the spinal column.

Fluorine is present in the soil and water as a naturally-occurring fluoride. The concentrations of fluoride in the soil or water is not the determinant of fluoride intake, but it is the total fluoride ingested—concentration times amount—that is important.

NUTRIENTS AND FOOD

Nutrient requirements or recommendations as established by various agencies and institutions provide guidelines for assessing the adequacy of dietary intakes on the population level. Inadequate or excessive intakes of either calories or specific nutrients may lead to nutritional disease, as may the presence of metabolic disturbances or disease states. The recognition of nutritional disease provides another method for assessing the nutritional adequacy of a population's diet.

Examination of the actual food consumed by a population is an important part of nutritional analysis. In order to do this, the basic nutrient composition of foods and the nutritional changes that occur in foods before consumption must be understood.

Filling nutritional requirements requires a large portion of any population's time and energy. From the resources available, a human group, generally through a process of trial and error, selects food items for its diet that will allow successful growth and maintenance of its members. Processing and preservation will be practiced that extracts the optimal nutrient value from the selected foods. The success of a population in selecting and processing foods determines in large part the health of that group.

Filling Dietary Requirements 4

Human nutrient requirements can be met from a wide variety of diets. No single combination of foods can be considered optimal. In each ecological zone, a number of food sources will be found, and from these are chosen a combination of items which will fill the inhabitants' requirements for energy, and for proteins and minerals.

ENERGY

Food energy is used by the body for maintaining basal metabolism, for growth, for reproduction, for temperature regulation, and for physical activity. About two-thirds of our daily energy requirement is taken up by basic life-support needs, such as heartbeat, blood circulation, breathing, and other body functions. The remainder supports our physical activity level. Energy released from food by oxidation is either used by the body, or it is stored as fat against a period of scarce resources.

The energy value of food is measured in terms of calories of heat released by its combustion. A calorie is defined as the amount of heat required to raise the temperature of one gram of water one degree centigrade. The caloric value used most often is kilocalorie. One kilocalorie (kcal) equals one thousand calories, and is defined as the amount of heat required to raise one kilogram of water one degree centigrade.

Calories used for energy can be obtained from carbohydrates, lipids (fats), proteins, and alcohol. The calories available from individual carbohydrates, proteins, lipids, and alcohol differ in their concentration. The gross energy yield (heat of combustion) of carbohydrates varies from 3.96 kcal per gm derived from sucrose, to 4.23 kcal per gm from starch, with an average carbohydrate energy yield of 4.15 kcal per gm. Lipids generally yield the highest energy value. Butterfat, for example, yields 9.21 kcal per gm and lard, 9.48 kcal per gm. The average yield of fats is generally given as 9.4 kcal per gm. Proteins yield intermediate energy values around 5.65 kcal per gm and alcohol yields roughly 7 kcal per gm (Pike & Brown, 1967).

The gross energy value of foodstuffs as measured by combustion does not represent the energy actually available to the body. Because no food is completely absorbed, potential energy is lost and never enters the tissues; rather, it is excreted in the feces. Of the major food items, on an average, 97% of ingested carbohydrates, 95% of fats, and 92% of proteins, are absorbed. The digestible energy value of foodstuffs is lower than the heat of combustion.

In addition, the energy value of proteins is further reduced because the cell is less efficient in oxidizing protein than carbohydrates and fats. Urea, uric acid, creatinine, and other nitrogenous compounds derived from proteins are excreted in the urine. After subtracting the caloric value of nitrogen lost in the urine, the "digestible" energy value of protein is 4 kcal per gm, the same as that for carbohydrates.

When heat of combustion is corrected for losses in digestion and for unmetabolized urinary losses, the energy value of foods is designated as available energy, or physiological fuel value. Available energy of the major foodstuffs is shown in Figure 4.1.

The energy value of a particular food depends on its contents of each of the calorie-containing components. Foods high in fat content (such as many meats and cheeses) or those low in water content (such as dried beans) are generally concentrated sources of calories. Foods low in fat and high in water content (such as leafy vegetables and most fresh fruit) are poor sources of calories.

NUTRIENT COMPONENTS OF FOODS

The specific nutrient components of food are listed in food composition tables which aid in estimating the availability of nutrients from food. No table is suitable for the accurate estimation of the nutrients in an individual diet, but they can be of use in calculating the approximate value of diets of populations.

Traditionally, tables of food composition have included data on energy,

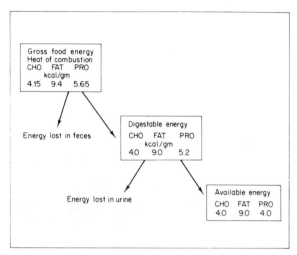

Figure 4-1. Available energy of foodstuffs. From Pike, R., and Brown, M. *Nutrition: An integrated approach,* John Wiley and Sons, Inc., 1967, p. 359.

approximate composition (water, crude protein, crude fat, crude fiber, and mineral ash), and the minerals and vitamins for which the National Research Council has made recommended dietary allowances. The trend now is toward more detailed identification of the nutrients present in foods, including, at times, sodium, potassium, copper, sulfur, and chloride content (Watt and Merrill 1963, Widdowson and McChance 1960).

CARBOHYDRATES, FATS, AND PROTEINS

Carbohydrates, fats, and proteins can all be used by the body as sources of energy, and amounts ingested in excess of caloric requirements can be stored as fat. In addition, the body muscles also represent a storehouse of protein. Protein constitutes 75% of the dry weight of soft tissue of the body. During periods of inadequate caloric intake, stored body fat and a certain amount of tissue protein can be broken down and converted into energy. The amount of body protein available for this purpose, however, is limited, and the cost to the organism can be great.

Fat differs from protein in that it can be stored in practically unlimited amounts. When food is ingested in excess of caloric needs, whether ingested as carbohydrates, fat, or protein, the equivalent of the excess calories is deposited as fat in the adipose tissues. When food intake is inadequate to meet caloric needs, fat is mobilized to make up the caloric deficit. In this way, practically the entire fat stores of the body can be depleted without severe consequences.

CARBOHYDRATES

The importance of carbohydrates as an energy source in human nutrition has varied greatly at different times and in different places. Grains, fruit, and vegetables are high in carbohydrate content, whereas meat, fish, and dairy products are not. Tropical diets often contain a proportionately high carbohydrate content, whereas those of the arctic regions traditionally have had a low carbohydrate proportion.

Although there has been some change in the food sources from which carbohydrates are derived, the proportion of carbohydrates in the United

TABLE 4.1
Types and Sources of Carbohydrates in the North American Diet

Carbohydrates	Approximate percentage of total CHO	Chief food sources
Polysaccharides	.	
Indigestible		
Cellulose	3	Stalks and leaves of vegetables
Hemicellulose		Outer seed covers
Pectins		Fruits
Partially Digestible	2	
Insulin		Jerusalem artichokes, onions
Galactogens		Snails
Mannosans		Legumes
Raffinose		Sugar beets
Pentosans		Fruits, gums
Digestible		
Starch & dextrins	50	Grains, vegetables
Glycogen	negligible	Meat, seafoods
Disaccharides		
Sucrose	25	Sugar, molasses, maple syrup
Lactose	10	Milk, milk products
Maltose	negligible	Malt products
Monosaccharides		
Hexoses		
Glucose	5	Fruits, honey, corn syrup
Fructose	5	Fruits, honey
Galactose	0	
Mannose	0	
Pentoses		
Ribose	0	Do not normally occur in free
Xylose	0	form in food
Arabinose	0	

SOURCE: Adapted from Soskin and Levine. In Wohl and Goodhart (eds.), *Modern nutrition in health and disease,* Lea and Febiger, 1955, p. 144.

States dietary has remained at about 50–60% of the total caloric intake (Soskin and Levine 1955). Table 4.1 shows the relative amounts and sources of carbohydrates in the North American diet.

Starch, sucrose, and lactose contribute the majority of carbohydrate calories in our diet, although in many parts of the world the starch contribution alone to the diet may reach 75–80% due to the consumption of large quantities of grain (rice, wheat, corn), or tubers (potatoes, manioc). The intake of lactose from milk and unfermented milk products, which is about 10% of the carbohydrates in the North American diet, may be insignificant in some regions.

LIPIDS

The lipids, which include both fats and oils, form the most concentrated source of food energy. The proportion of total dietary calories from fats varies widely from population to population. Lipids accounted for at least 30% of North American and German diets between 1926 and 1930 (Deuel 1955). Since then, the consumption of fats has increased in this country and now comprises about 40% of the total dietary calories, of which two-thirds comes from animal and one-third from vegetable sources (Kromer 1961). Most of the increase is due to a greater consumption of animal products and seems to be characteristic of most Western countries. The trend in visible fat consumption has been toward greater consumption of margarine, shortening, and oil, and decreased consumption of butter and lard. The traditional Japanese diet, on the other hand, provides only 10% of the total calories in the form of lipids (Brandt 1943).

Lipids can be found in both plant and animal sources. Those fats having lower melting points and which are commonly found in the liquid stage usually have a larger proportion of unsaturated fatty acids than fats with higher melting points and which are consequently usually found in the solid state.

Table 4.2 lists the forms in which lipids are found in nature. Within the lipids fats and oils comprise the largest group. The value of lipids in the diet usually is that of a concentrated source of calories. Fats are also carriers of the fat-soluble vitamins: vitamin A, vitamin D, vitamin K, and the tocopherols (vitamin E). In addition, the lipids include the essential fatty acids which are polyunsaturated fats necessary for normal nutrition and which cannot be produced by human tissues. The three acids included in this category are linoleic acid, linolenic acid, and arachidonic acid. Current practice is to consider only linoleic acid as significant in human dietaries. The requirement for linoleic acid has been demonstrated for normal growth in human infants, but the dietary requirement for the human adult appears

TABLE 4.2
Classification of Lipids

Simple lipids
   Neutral fats—glycerol esters of fatty acids
   Waxes
     True waxes
     Cholesterol esters
     Vitamin A esters
     Vitamin D esters
Compound or conjugate lipids
   Phospholipids—contain orthophophate molecule
   Cerebrosides—contain carbohydrate molecule
   Sulfolipids—contain sulfate group
   Gangliosides—related to cerebrosides, occur in ganglion cells
   Lipoproteins—lipids bound to proteins
Derived lipids
   Fatty acids
   Alcohols
   Hydrocarbons
   Vitamins D
   Vitamins E
   Vitamins K

SOURCE: Adapted from Alfin-Slater and Deuel. In Wohl and Goodhart (eds.), *Modern nutrition in health and disease,* Lea and Febiger, 1960, pp. 173–175.

to be negligible because apparently tissue stores of essential fatty acid in the adult are high.

PROTEINS

Protein can be metabolized and converted into calories by the human body. However, when sufficient calories are provided by lipids and carbohydrates, proteins are broken down into their constituent parts and are converted into body tissue and the precursors of compounds required in metabolic processes.

Dietary protein is derived from both animal and vegetable sources. The protein content of different food substances varies considerably, as demonstrated in Table 4.3.

Traditional Western diets contain an average of 14% of total calories in the form of protein, and only rarely do calories from protein fall below 10% of total calories (USDA 1953). The protein in a daily average U.S. diet of 2500 calories is about 94 gm. In contrast to the Western diet, the food in some lesser-industrialized countries, where primarily starches, roots, vegetables, and fruits are consumed, contains much lower concentrations of protein.

A protein is a polymer of amino acids joined by peptide bonds. Although the range of structure and complexity is great, the molecular weight of a protein is usually high. The amino acids present, their position in the molecule, and the spatial arrangement of the molecule all determine the properties and characteristics of the protein.

Some of the amino acids required for protein synthesis in growth, repair, and maintenance must be supplied by ingested food, but others may be produced by the body itself. The amino acids which must be supplied by the diet are called "essential." They are no more important in growth or metabolism than the others, but only require a supply from external sources. The essential and nonessential amino acids are listed in Table 3.6.

TABLE 4.3
Protein Content of Some Common Foods

Food	Kilocalories per 100 grams	Grams of protein per 100 grams	Percentage protein kilocalories of total kilocalories
Pork meat (cooked, medium fat)	457	14.9	13.9
Beef (cooked, medium fat)	273	17.5	27.4
Chicken meat (total edible)	302	18.0	25.5
Fish fillet (unspecific)	132	18.8	60.7
Canned tuna (in oil)	217	27.7	54.4
Salmon, canned	173	20.2	49.9
Eggs, fresh	144	11.0	33.3
Milk, whole	68	3.5	22.0
Skim milk, dry	360	36.0	42.7
Cheese, hard	341	34.0	42.6
Whey cheese (soft)	106	14.0	56.4
Rice, raw (white)	360	6.7	7.1
Rice, cooked (white)	109	2.0	7.3
Cornmeal (whole ground)	356	9.3	10.0
Wheat flour (medium extraction)	350	11.7	13.0
Potatoes, raw	70	1.7	6.7
Beans, peas (dry)	345	22.2	22.3
Cabbage, fresh	11	1.1	24.4
Fruit, fresh (unspecified)	46	0.5	3.6

SOURCE: Adapted from Geiger. In Wohl and Goodhart (eds.), *Modern nutrition in health and disease,* Lea and Febiger, 1955, p. 100.

If any one of the essential amino acids is missing from the diet, or is present in inadequate quantities, the dietary protein cannot be used for growth and maintenance, even though the other amino acids may be present in abundance. A shortage in one of the nonessential amino acids can be corrected by producing it in the body from other sources.

The pattern of amino acids best utilized for human growth and maintenance has been established as an indicator of protein quality. Those foods containing amino acids in the proportions best utilized by the human body are said to contain "high-quality" proteins.

With the exception of gelatin, proteins from animal sources (meat, fish, milk, and eggs) are of high quality. Soybean protein is roughly equivalent to most animal proteins, but the rest of the vegetable or grain proteins are low in some essential amino acid such as lysine, tryptophan, threonine, or methionine. When eaten alone, a vegetable or grain protein would not promote satisfactory growth. Most diets, however, contain a mixture of different proteins, with a variety of amino acid patterns such as those present in grains, legumes, and vegetables. It is the total of all amino acids consumed that determines the biological value of the dietary protein, not the sum of the quality of each protein consumed individually.

Traditionally, each human population has, from the foods available, created a diet containing foods with complementary amino-acid patterns. The traditional Native American diet of corn, beans, and squash, or the tropical American diet of rice, beans, and chiles, creates a total diet of high protein quality, even though each individual food item contains an incomplete protein. It is not absolutely necessary to eat high-quality proteins such as fish, meat, eggs, or milk for maintenance of growth and good health. Entire populations, living on strictly vegetarian diets, do not necessarily suffer from protein deficiency because the combinations of foods which comprise their diet are able to fill their amino-acid requirements.

It must be emphasized that effective amino-acid supplementation occurs only when the different and supplementary proteins are eaten simultaneously or within a short interval of time of each other.

MINERALS AND VITAMINS

The requirements for minerals and vitamins are minor compared to the large amounts of calories and protein required by the body. While requirements for some minerals may be comparatively large, in the range of one gram, the vitamin requirements are small, and may be measured in micrograms. In addition to the small amounts being considered, the study of dietary vitamins and minerals is made even more difficult by problems of absorption, of complex interrelationships between nutrients, and of nutrient losses during food processing and preparation.

MINERALS

The minerals that are present in fairly large quantities in the human body and known to be essential are calcium, phosphorus, potassium, sodium, chloride, magnesium, and sulfur.

Magnesium

Magnesium deficiency does not appear to be a problem in most human diets since the mineral is widely distributed in foods. In a normally adequate diet, about 30% of the total magnesium may come from green vegetables that contain the magnesium porphyrin, chlorophyll. Magnesium deficiency may occur in humans as a result of prolonged episodes of vomiting or malabsorption as occurs with severe diarrhea. Magnesium deficiency has been reported in children with protein-calorie malnutrition, due primarily to diarrhea which increases fecal loss of the mineral (Caddell 1969).

Sodium

Dietary deficiencies of sodium probably never occur in humans, since human diets generally contain more sodium than necessary. Sodium is widely distributed in foodstuffs. Plant sources contain less than animal products, and processed foods of all kinds tend to have a high sodium content, since many sodium compounds are used to preserve, tenderize, and flavor. Intakes also vary widely; about 10 gm of sodium chloride daily appears to be usual for most North Americans, whereas intakes of 30–40 gm daily are not uncommon in Asian countries where soy sauces and monosodium glutamate are used for flavoring (Pike and Brown, 1967).

Chloride

The chloride ion, the major anion of the extracellular fluid, occurs, for the most part, in combination with sodium. In normal individuals, dietary chloride intake is of little practical significance.

Potassium

Potassium, the chief cation of the intracellular fluid, is necessary for carbohydrate and protein metabolism. A deficiency of potassium is unlikely to occur as a result of dietary lack. Body potassium may be depleted by excessive excretion through the kidneys or through the gastrointestinal tract.

Sulfur

The bulk of the sulfur present in the human body is derived from the three sulfur-containing amino acids: methionine, cystine, and cysteine, which provide the sulfur needed for synthesis of other sulfur-containing compounds. As long as these amino acids are present in the diet in sufficient quantities, no other dietary source of sulfur is required.

Calcium and Phosphorus

Calcium and phosphorus are usually considered together as they constitute the major part of the mineral content of the human skeleton. Most of the body's calcium and phosphorus are contained in the bones, and the ratio of calcium to phosphorus, while not entirely constant, is nearly so.

The bones constitute a mineral reserve which may be drawn on in time of inadequate calcium intake. The more easily mobilized calcium in trabeculae (spongy bone) is of particular importance during pregnancy and lactation when calcium requirements are very high.

It is obvious that the nutritional requirements for calcium and phosphorus are related to bone formation in the growing child and the fetus, and to milk production in the adult female. Bone growth and maintenance are not solely a matter of calcium and phosphorus metabolism, however. In addition to the more apparent contributions of protein to bone matrix formation and vitamin D to mineralization are the effects of vitamin A, magnesium, and vitamin C.

Despite considerable individual differences, humans utilize calcium rather inefficiently. As little as 20–30% of dietary calcium may be absorbed. Many factors influence actual absorption. Generally, the body utilizes nutrients more efficiently when in need, and calcium is no exception.

The ratio of calcium or phosphorus in the diet may also play a role in absorption. A dietary calcium–phosphorus ratio of about 1:1 is ideal. Absorption of both calcium and phosphorus is reduced by the presence of high levels of phytic acid in the diet. Much of the phosphorus in cereals occurs as phytic acid. Formation of relatively insoluble calcium phytate in the gut decreases the supply of both phosphorus and calcium. Diets very high in whole wheat may produce fecal calcium losses in excess of dietary calcium intake.

Oxalates form insoluble salts which also render calcium unavailable to the body. A few vegetables such as rhubarb and spinach contain oxalic acid in excess of their calcium content.

Calcium absorption is favored in turn by a low intestinal pH. Good calcium absorption from consuming lactose (milk sugar) may be due to lactic-acid fermentation which increases acidity in the gut. Hydrochloric acid in the stomach is of importance as well, because it increases stomach acidity, and, therefore, aids in calcium absorption.

Both plant and animal products may be valuable sources of calcium and phosphorus. In Table 4.4 are some average values for the calcium and phosphorus content of various foods. Most common foods, other than milk and green leafy vegetables, contain considerably more phosphorus than calcium, thus accounting for the greater interest in calcium in human nutrition.

The milk products which have traditionally been an important source of dietary calcium in Western diets may be scarce in the diets of other populations. In those cases, the low concentration of calcium present in foods which are ingested in large quantities, such as greens or beans, are of primary importance. It may also be that unusual calcium sources are playing an important role in the diet. For example, the ingestion of small fish or chicken bones will be sufficient to fill dietary calcium requirements when this occurs on a regular basis.

TABLE 4.4
Average Calcium and Phosphorus Content of Selected Foods

Food	Calcium mg per 100 gm	Phosphorus mg per 100 gm
Cow's milk	118	93
Human milk	32	13
Beef	11	170
Pork	7	117
Beans, dry	163	437
Peas, dry mature	57	388
Potatoes	11	56
Sweet potatoes	30	49
Carrots	39	37
White bread (4% nonfat milk solids)	79	92
White bread (no milk solids)	13	77
Corn meal	6	99
Oatmeal	55	405
Cabbage	46	31
Kale	225	62
Lettuce	22	25
Apples	6	10
Grapefruit	22	18
Peaches	8	22
Brazil nuts	186	693
Peanuts	74	393

SOURCE: From Hegsted. In Wohl and Goodhart (eds.), *Modern nutrition in health and disease*, Lea and Febiger, 1955, p. 217.

IRON AND THE ESSENTIAL TRACE ELEMENTS

Six of the elements found in human tissues in minute amounts are known to be essential: copper, cobalt, molybdenum, iodine, manganese, and zinc. Iron is needed in larger quantities and cannot properly be classified as a trace element. While traces of other minerals are also frequently found in tissue, there is no convincing evidence that they are necessary to life.

Proof that any element is essential to life depends largely on the demonstration that when it is deficient, certain signs or metabolic defects result, and that the abnormalities can be corrected by replacement therapy of that mineral. Experiments on animals have provided these criteria for copper, manganese, and zinc. The amounts of cobalt needed by the human body are so minute that no laboratory diet has been prepared capable of producing cobalt deficiency.

In human populations, depletion of cobalt, manganese, and molybdenum of a magnitude sufficient to cause health problems, has not been recognized. Copper deficiencies have been demonstrated in infants maintained for long periods of time on milk alone (Cordano, Baertl, and Graham 1964).

Simple goiter, associated often, but not always, with a deficiency of iodine, is endemic in many areas of the world. Iodine content of foods varies widely, depending upon the iodine content of the soil and water in which food was grown. The seeds and edible portions of most crucifera (cabbage, turnips, rutabagas) contain a compound that can induce goiters in experimental animals fed large amounts of the food. While it is doubtful that humans could consume enough of any potentially goitrogenic foods to seriously affect thyroid activity, it is possible that goitrogenic foods may accentuate the effects of low iodine intake and contribute to the formation of goiters.

Iron

Iron, as an essential component of the molecular structure of hemoglobin, myoglobin, the cytochromes, and other enzyme systems, is required for oxygen transport and cellular respiration. The intestinal mucosa serves to some extent as a regulator of iron balance. Iron is absorbed more efficiently by people with iron deficiency or hypochromic anemia than by normal subjects. Ascorbic acid (vitamin C) and foods containing ascorbic acid enhance iron absorption.

The diet of healthy adults in the United States contains about 12–15 mg of iron per day. Using this figure as the basis for calculation, the amount of iron absorbed from food each day probably varies from .6 to 1.5 mg. Poor diet, steatorrhea, or diarrhea decreases the amount even further (Moore 1955).

Most assimilated iron is used for the daily synthesis of hemoglobin. Only a fraction of the iron required for hemoglobin synthesis is ingested each day. The remainder comes from body stores, or from iron salvage when erythrocytes and other cells are destroyed.

Several factors are known to influence the utilization of iron for hemoglobin synthesis. Infection causes iron to be diverted from plasma to the liver and other tissues. Copper is required in order for iron to be used to build hemoglobin. Approximately 1 gram of iron, in the form of feritin and hemosiderin, is stored in the tissues of adults, primarily in the liver and spleen. The iron can be mobilized by the body when the need exists.

Because of the relatively high iron requirements of growing children and premenopausal women, an adequate dietary intake is necessary to maintain a positive iron balance. Infants fed a low-iron milk diet without supplementation after the first six months of life have a high incidence of iron deficiency. Famines or food shortages cause a striking increase in hypochromic anemia among women and children.

The recommended dietary allowances (Table 3.2) of 10–15 mg of iron for infants and young children, and 18 mg for adult females, can hardly be supplied by the usual United States diets. Typical North American diets contain about 6 mg of iron per 1000 kcal; thus an adult woman could reasonably be expected to consume roughly 12 gm of iron per day. Infants consuming only milk, a poor source of iron, would have access to negligible amounts of iron without supplementation. Most North Americans derive their iron from dietary meats and eggs. As can be seen in Table 4.5, seeds, nuts, and beans are also good iron sources.

VITAMINS

Vitamins are chemically unrelated organic substances essential in the human diet in minute amounts required for specific metabolic reactions. Traditionally, vitamins are classified according to their solubility in either water or fat and fat solvents. This property determines patterns of transport, excretion, and storage within the human body. Historically, vitamins were discovered by their absence in the diet and the resultant clinical syndromes or symptoms characteristic of the particular vitamin-deficiency state.

Water-Soluble Vitamins

Thiamine Classical beri-beri, the thiamine deficiency disease, is rarely seen in Europe and North America, except as caused by alcoholism or conditions of extreme poverty where negligible amounts of thiamine are consumed. Meatless diets based on highly refined grains, such as polished

TABLE 4.5
Iron Content of Common Foods[a]

Food	Iron mg per 100 gm
Chicken (white meat, cooked)	1.3
Beef, (ground, cooked)	3.2
Liver (beef, cooked)	8.8
Egg (fried)	2.4
Codfish (cooked)	1.0
Clams (raw)	6.1
Spinach (canned)	9.5
Bread (white, enriched)	2.5
Corn flour	1.8
Beans (red, cooked)	2.4
Beans (lima, cooked)	2.5
Peanuts (roasted, shelled)	10.0
Sunflower seeds (hulled)	32.2
Carrots (cooked)	.6
Apple (fresh)	.3
Milk (whole, cow's)	.2

[a]Values taken from Watt and Merrill 1963.

rice or milled corn, are most commonly associated with thiamine deficiency. Additionally, there is an enzyme in raw carp and raw herring, called thiaminase, which can cause rapid destruction of thiamine activity when the raw fish is mixed in the diet.

The richest dietary sources of thiamine are pork, liver, yeast, whole cereals, and fresh green vegetables. Many foodstuffs lose much of their thiamine content during cooking and serving. There is little thiamine inactivation in foods heated in acid or neutral solutions at 100°C, but higher temperatures and increased alkalinity hasten the rate of thiamine destruction. Freezing causes little or no loss in thiamine content of foods.

Riboflavin The first descriptions of riboflavin deficiency were based on observations from Ceylon, Jamaica, West Africa, Singapore, South India, and the United States (Horwitt 1955). Riboflavin hypovitaminosis is still widespread, and it is not difficult to construct a riboflavin-deficient diet by omitting dairy foods and other animal-protein sources.

Riboflavin is relatively heat-stable in the absence of light, which favors its preservation in ordinary cooking techniques. The major losses that may occur are attributed to the extraction of riboflavin by the cooking water used for boiling or blanching (Mickelsen and Makdani 1975).

Niacin   Niacin (nicotinic acid) is the human antipellagric vitamin. Pellagra has been endemic in corn-eating populations for over 200 years. The need for dietary niacin cannot be separated from the tryptophan content of the diet. In general, most animal-protein foods are high in tryptophan. Liver, meats, dried yeast, and wheat bran are good sources of both tryptophan and niacin.

Whole corn, so often associated with pellagra, is not limited in its niacin content, but is quite low in tryptophan. A niacin-deficient diet is generally one containing a high proportion of cereal products, and, for practical purposes, pellagra remains a disease associated with maize-eating populations.

Pantothenic Acid   Pantothenic acid plays an important role in normal adrenocortical function. It is doubtful that pantothenic-acid deficiency occurs except in the most unusual circumstances, or as a result of excessive metabolic demands. Pantothenic acid is widely distributed in nature, a property from which its name is derived. Liver, meat, cereal, and milk are all reliable sources of the vitamin. Pantothenic acid can be synthesized by bacteria and it is thought that human gastroenteric-tract organisms provide a considerable amount to the host.

Vitamin B$_6$ Group   Pyridoxine, pyridoxal, pyridoxamine, and pyridoxal phosphate form the vitamin B$_6$ group. Vitamin B$_6$ occurs in animal products, largely in its pyridoxal and pyridoxamine forms, while pyridoxine is the largest vitamin B$_6$ component in vegetable foods. An additional vitamin B$_6$ source available to humans may be that synthesized by the intestinal organisms.

The widespread availability of pyridoxine in natural foods, the possibility of gastrointestinal-tract bacterial synthesis of the vitamin, or the similarity of the lesions of vitamin B$_6$ deficiency to those of the mixed B-complex deficiency state, may explain why pyridoxine deficiency is so seldom recognized under natural conditions in humans.

Folic Acid   Folic acid occurs widely distributed in nature. Deep-green leafy vegetables and liver are both rich in folic acid. An average human diet selected from a wide variety of foods, supplies .5–1.0 mg of folic-acid compounds daily, most of it in conjugated form that must be broken down in the body by enzyme systems found in the tissues. It is probable that at least some folic acid is obtained by the human host from intestinal microorganisms. Folic- or folinic-acid deficiency states have not been induced in human beings.

Vitamin B₁₂   Vitamin B_{12} may exist in several different forms, which have been given the generic name cobalamine. Much of the vitamin B_{12} in food occurs in the form of a protein complex. Such bound forms are inactive for the growth of most microorganisms until the vitamin B_{12} moiety is released by protoeolytic enzymes or heat. Vitamin B_{12} is found almost exclusively in foods of animal origin, although it is synthesized by many bacteria. It is probable, however, that little of the vitamin derived from gastrointestinal tract organisms is available to the human host.

In general, the best sources of vitamin B_{12} are liver, kidneys, meat, and milk. Over 70% of vitamin B_{12} is retained during cooking.

Vitamin B_{12}, released from its combination with food protein in the stomach and upper gastroenteric tract, requires the presence of an "intrinsic factor" for its absorption. Individuals suffering from pernicious anemia develop the disease because they are deficient in intrinsic factor, and this leads to vitamin B_{12} deficiency.

Vitamin C (ascorbic acid)   Ascorbic acid is a substance of great physiological importance because of its involvement in a large number of intracellular chemical reactions. The only significant dietary sources of ascorbic acid are fruits, vegetables, and liver. Meats, cereals, and dairy products contain such small amounts that they are usually of little importance as dietary sources of vitamin C. Other vitamin C sources, less common to the North American diet, include green walnuts, rose hips, pine needles, and guava.

Fat-Soluble Vitamins

Vitamin A   Vitamin A occurs only in animal organisms. The most abundant food sources of vitamin A are milk, butter, egg yolks, liver, and kidney. In addition, various fish liver oils are excellent sources. The vitamin A precursor, carotene, is the chief source of vitamin A in most diets. Carotene is converted to vitamin A in the intestinal wall during absorption. Dietary carotene has about half the biological activity of preformed vitamin A. This may be because vitamin A is more readily absorbed from the intestine than carotene, or because carotene is not efficiently converted to vitamin A. Sources of carotene are the green leaves of plants, cabbage, carrots, lettuce, spinach, tomatoes, and alfalfa.

While vitamin A is readily destroyed by oxidation, it is heat stable, and both vitamin A and carotene are able to withstand common processes of cooking and boiling. Drastic or prolonged heating and dehydration will cause oxidation which destroys the vitamin.

Vitamin D There are a number of substances which possess vitamin D activity, the most important of which are vitamin D_2 (calciferol) and vitamin D_3. Vitamin D_3 is the naturally occurring substance found in egg yolk, butter, and fish liver oils. Under the influence of ultraviolet radiation, it is formed from provitamin D_3 which is present in the surface of the skin. Ingested vitamin D is absorbed with food fats and any condition that interferes with fat absorption also interferes with the absorption of vitamin D.

Vitamin K Vitamin K, the antihemorrhagic vitamin, is widely distributed in nature. It is found principally in leafy vegetables and is especially plentiful in alfalfa. It is found in traces in cereals and animal tissues. Vitamin K can be synthesized by many bacteria, including those normally present in the human intestine. Under most circumstances the bacterial flora of the intestine provide an adequate supply of vitamin K in humans. An adequate supply of bile salts is necessary for absorption of the vitamin from the small intestine.

Vitamin E The tocopherols, generally referred to collectively as vitamin E, occur principally in plant oils and are especially abundant in wheat germ oils. Vitamin E is also present in corn oil, cottonseed oil, lettuce, and alfalfa. There is very little in cow's milk, but mature human milk contains 2 to 4 times as much as cow's milk, and human colostrum up to 20 times as much vitamin E as cow's milk.

It is present in animal tissues, principally in fat and muscles, but not in high concentrations. The tocopherols are stable to heat in the absence of oxygen. Ultraviolet radiation destroys the vitamin activity as does oxidation.

NUTRITIONAL CONSEQUENCES OF FOOD PROCESSING

From the time of harvest or slaughter, raw plant and animal tissues undergo gradual deterioration by various biological forces. The major causes of food deterioration are microbial growth, enzyme action, and chemical changes. The rate of deterioration varies, depending on the water content of the tissues, temperature, pH, and other environmental factors. Nutrients in food continue to be destroyed when foods are processed prior to consumption because nutrients are sensitive to the pH of the solvent, oxygen, light, and heat, or combinations of these. Trace elements, especially copper and iron, and enzymes may catalyze these effects. Nutrient stability under various conditions is summarized in Table 4.6.

TABLE 4.6
Nutrient Stability

	Effect of pH						
Nutrient	Neutral pH 7	Acid <pH 7	Alkaline >pH 7	Air or oxygen	Light	Heat	Max cooking losses
Vitamins							%
Vitamin A	S	U	S	U	U	U	40
Ascorbic acid (C)	U	S	U	U	U	U	100
Biotin	S	S	S	S	S	U	60
Carotene (pro-A)	S	U	S	U'	U	U	30
Choline	S	S	S	U	S	S	5
Cobalamin (B-12)	S	S	S	U	U	S	10
Vitamin D	S		U	U	U	U	40
Folic acid	U	U	S	U	U	U	100
Inositol	S	S	S	S	S	U	95
Vitamin K	S	U	U	S	U	S	5
Niacin (PP)	S	S	S	S	S	S	75
Pantothenic acid	S	U	U	S	S	U	50
p-Amino benzoic acid	S	S	S	U	S	S	5
Pyridoxine (B-6)	S	S	S	S	U	U	40
Riboflavin (B-2)	S	S	U	S	U	U	75
Thiamin (B-1)	U	S	U	U	S	U	80
Tocopherol (E)	S	S	S	U	U	U	55
Essential amino acids							
Isoleucine	S	S	S	S	S	S	10
Leucine	S	S	S	S	S	S	10
Lysine	S	S	S	S	S	U	40
Methionine	S	S	S	S	S	S	10
Phenylalanine	S	S	S	S	S	S	5
Threonine	S	U	U	S	S	U	20
Tryptophan	S	U	S	S	U	S	15
Valine	S	S	S	S	S	S	10
Essential fatty acids	S	S	U	U	U	S	10
Mineral salts	S	S	S	S	S	S	3

SOURCE: Data from Harris. In Harris and Karmas, *Nutritional evaluation of food processing*, 2nd ed. AVI Pub. Co., P.O. Box 831, Westport, Conn. 06880.
S = stable (no important destruction).
U = unstable (significant destruction).

EFFECTS OF STORAGE AND HANDLING

Foods of plant and animal origin vary in their nutrient content and in their susceptibility to various biological forces. Consequently their nutrient losses during storage and handling vary greatly.

When fruits and vegetables are harvested and stored prior to processing, chemical changes continue which result in gradual decline in nutritional quality. Moisture loss, which begins as soon as a fruit or vegetable is harvested, can cause nutritive loss. The rate of moisture loss depends on the extent and the nature of the surface area of the product and upon the temperature and humidity of the environment. Leafy vegetables, because of their extensive and relatively permeable surfaces, wilt and lose vitamin C and carotene when transported or stored at high temperatures and/or low humidities, with temperature having the more severe effect (Krochta and Feinberg, 1975). Root vegetables, tightly packed heads of cabbage, and hard fruit lose vitamin C more slowly, retaining some of the original vitamin content even after 6 months of storage.

Seeds in a dormant condition, put into storage until needed, are remarkably resistant to deterioration. The storage ability of seeds usually correlates with their life span (Frampton, 1975). Short-lived species remain viable under good storage conditions for about 3 years, while long-lived seeds may remain viable for up to 100 years.

The main danger to stored seed is attack by insects and fungi. Although the seed coats are protective, they may suffer physical damage by insects and other pests, or by rough handling during harvesting, making them more susceptible to attack. The storage of damp seeds and poor storage conditions also contribute to seed loss. Dampness and warm storage temperatures both hasten the growth of insects and fungi.

Among the factors which must be controlled to avoid deterioration of stored seed are the moisture, both of the seed itself and the ambient atmosphere, the storage temperature, the maturity of seed going into storage, destruction by insects, fungi, and other pests, and the handling of seed during harvest (Frampton, 1975).

Foods of animal origin, with the possible exception of shell eggs, are subject to prompt bacterial attack and to oxidative changes in fatty portions exposed to air unless some method of preservation is used. Refrigeration during storage and shipment minimizes nutrient changes.

Surface dehydration and loss of tissue fluid from cut surfaces reduces the weight of meats but does not markedly affect nutrient content since removal of moisture only concentrates the solids of meats and does not change their total quantity. The amount of fluid loss is influenced by the rate of ambient air movement and humidity. High humidity, while reducing moisture loss, increases the tendency for bacterial and mold growth. Except for small losses of niacin, vitamin content of meat remains stable until spoilage occurs, and there does not seem to be significant protein destruction. Amino acid stability is assumed (Rice, 1975).

Fish on the other hand is subject to rapid spoilage due both to bacterial and autolytic changes which lead to increases in the amounts of free amino acids and polypeptides and later, secondary decomposition. It is doubtful however that significant nutrient loss occurs before spoilage.

Milk is readily attacked by bacteria, but except for a very rapid loss of vitamin C, the nutrients of milk are stable during normal periods of storage. If milk is exposed to sunlight or to strong light, riboflavin is also destroyed.

Evaporation of moisture from shell eggs occurs proportionately with the time of storage. At high temperature or at low humidity, greater losses occur. Folic acid and vitamin B_6 are the only two vitamins showing marked decrease during storage (Rice, 1975).

EFFECTS OF FOOD PRESERVATION

By manipulating environmental factors, food preservation techniques are employed to prevent nutrient losses through deterioration. There are five traditional food processing techniques for preservation. These are: (a) moisture removal (drying, dehydration, concentration), (b) heat treatment (blanching, pasteurization, sterilization), (c) low-temperature treatment (refrigeration, cooling, freezing), (d) acidity control (fermentation, acidic additives), and (e) processing additives (curing, salting, smoking) (Karmas, 1975).

Removal of biologically active water through drying or dehydration stops the growth of microorganisms and reduces the rate of enzyme activity and chemical reactions. The effect of water removal on nutritional change is relatively small if the dehydration temperature is moderate and the food adequately protected during storage.

The principal effect of heat treatment is the inactivation of enzymes by the denaturation of proteins. Heat sterilization, the most effective process of food preservation, has a severe effect on heat-labile nutrients, particularly vitamins, and reduces the nutritional quality of proteins.

Low-temperature preservation is the most harmless method of food preservation. Low temperature inhibits microbial growth and slows down the rate of chemical and enzyme reactions. Vitamin losses are minimal as compared with other methods of food preservation.

Anaerobic fermentation of carbohydrates produces lactic acid which lowers the pH of the food and inhibits the growth of food spoilage organisms. Acidity of foods may also be increased by acidic additives, such as vinegar or citric acid. Loss of nutrients through fermentation is small. In some cases the nutrient level may even be increased through microbial vitamin and protein synthesis.

The preservation of foods by chemical additives provides an inhibitory environment for microbial growth as well as enzyme and chemical reactions. Such processing may involve curing agents and smoking of flesh foods, high-sugar preservation of fruits and vegetables, and treatment with inhibiting chemical additives. The effect of these methods on nutrients is variable, but generally small (Karmas, 1975).

EFFECTS OF PROCESSING PRIOR TO CONSUMPTION

Whether food items are stored, preserved, or consumed soon after harvesting, some processing generally occurs prior to consumption. Nutrient losses occur in the trimming and discarding of meat and plant parts which are considered inedible or undesireable. This may include fat, skin, pits, or bruised spots. Obviously, the decision to trim is highly variable, and depends on custom and on economic factors.

For foods of animal origin, the losses of major interest are those from fat trim, while for foods of plant origin the losses are those from trimming, washing and soaking, and chopping. Fat trim is mostly fat with only small amounts of protein, from 2.1 to 4.5% (Lachance, 1975). Fat loss will also result in the loss of fat-soluble vitamins.

When foods of plant origin are trimmed, the nutrient losses generally exceed the weight losses, because nutrients are usually found in higher concentrations in the outer layers of seeds, tubers, roots, and fruits. Vitamin C is present in the highest concentrations just beneath the peel of the potato. The peel of carrots is especially rich in thiamin, niacin, and riboflavin, while the outer leaves of lettuce and spinach are rich in the B vitamins and in vitamin C. The outer green leaves are often richer in mineral salts. The leaves of many vegetables contain up to 6 times as much vitamin C as the stems, and more minerals as well (Lachance, 1975).

Preliminary washing and soaking of vegetables and tubers before cooking extracts water-soluble nutrients, but these losses are generally insignificant. The loss of vitamin C from chopped leafy vegetables can be considerable, up to 40%. Lesser vitamin C losses are also reported for other sliced fruits and vegetables.

During cooking, further nutrient losses may occur, depending on the amount of added water or fat used in cooking, and the temperature at which the food is cooked. Meats show losses of thiamin, riboflavin, niacin, and protein, with all cooking techniques. Protein losses are higher when water is added during cooking. Actual losses vary greatly with the cut of meat. Lower cooking temperatures result in greater retention of riboflavin, thiamin, niacin, and pantothenic acid. The retention of the heat-stable vitamins, riboflavin and niacin, are only slightly affected by high temperatures (Lachance, 1975).

When cooking food of plant origin, the greatest retention of vitamins A and C results from cooking without added water and the least retention is associated with cooking in the largest volume of water. Cooking by steaming above water retains as much as cooking in a small amount of water. Similar effects of water on cooking are demonstrated for the minerals, calcium, iron, and phosphorus, and the vitamins, thiamin, riboflavin, and niacin (Lachance, 1975). Solution losses in cooking are also affected by the amount of surface, especially cut surface, exposed to the water.

Special cooking and processing techniques may also be practiced to increase the nutrient content or nutrient availability of foods. The alkali treatment of corn is a well-known example from Central America. Maize, the largest source of calories and protein for many of the people of Central America, is limited in the quality and quantity of its essential amino acids and niacin. Alkali cooking techniques free otherwise unavailable nutrients in corn, allowing it to serve as a dietary staple (Katz, Hediger and Valleroy, 1974).

Corn is manufactured into tortillas by first heating the corn to almost boiling in a 5% solution of lime in water. The effect of the lime is to yield a dilute calcium hydroxide solution which is basic or alkaline. The lime treatment increases the nutritional quality of corn probably by causing a relative decrease in the solubility of the portion of the corn proteins which are deficient in lysine and tryptophan. The result is an increase in the relative amounts of lysine and tryptophan, and an increase in both the relative and absolute ratios of isoleucine to leucine. Other essential amino acids are also relatively doubled in concentration, and the availability of niacin and niacin precursors appear to be enhanced.

A deficiency of niacin and the niacin precursor tryptophan is associated with the deficiency disease pellagra. There is evidence to suggest that pellagra can also be induced by an unfavorable isoleucine to leucine ratio. Both niacin deficiency and an excessive amount of leucine, a leucine to isoleucine ratio nearly three times greater than that considered optimal, are found in a diet heavily dependent on corn. The alkali treatment of corn prior to consumption in the form of tortillas increases the overall nutritional quality of corn as a staple by increasing the relative isoleucine concentration and minimizing niacin deficiency.

A Middle Eastern example of food processing to enhance nutrient availability is the addition of a leavening agent to bread to reduce phytate binding of zinc. Bread, the main source of calories for many in the region, is made in some areas without leavening or fermentation. Bread consumed where zinc deficiency is not common is similar except that it has been allowed to ferment for several hours after a leavening agent has been added. The leavened bread contains considerably less phytate than unleavened bread, probably due to the destruction of phytate by the enzyme phytase produced by the yeast. Phytates are known to bind with various metal ions, including zinc, and prevent their absorption from the intestine. Fermentation of the bread may be sufficient to prevent zinc deficiency due to phytate binding in areas where zinc consumption would otherwise be adequate.

INTERFERENCE WITH THE USE OF INGESTED NUTRIENTS

Ingested nutrients may not contribute to the health of the organism if they are not absorbed from the gastrointestinal tract, or if they are bound in a nonfunctional compound. Failure to absorb or utilize nutrients may be the result of genetic malabsorption syndromes, disease states, or the presence of antimetabolites.

ANTIMETABOLITES

Certain specific chemicals are capable of reversing or blocking the effects of other related substances in biological systems. The compounds responsible for these blocking effects are termed "antimetabolites" because they prevent the utilization of normally-occurring nutrients by living tissues. Although a variety of antimetabolites have either been discovered or synthesized, few are of importance in the human diet. A comprehensive coverage of antimetabolites can be found in Woolley (1963) and Somogyi (1966).

AVIDIN

Eggwhite contains a specific protein "avidin," which combines with biotin and prevents this vitamin from entering the bloodstream when present in the intestinal tract. Avidin is denatured by heat, and its power of combining with biotin is limited. Biotin deficiency can be produced in human subjects by feeding them a diet in which approximately 30% of the total calories are supplied by dessicated eggwhite. Avidin is not an antimetabolite of biotin in a strict sense, but it induces the deficiency by interfering with the absorption of the vitamin from the gut.

GOITROGENS

Certain plants, particularly in the *Cruciferae*, but also including soybeans, contain substances which depress the uptake of iodine by the thyroid gland. The production of the thyroid hormone is subsequently diminished. It is unclear whether these goitrogens will by themselves produce signs of goiter, but they are thought to contribute to goiter in areas where iodine content of the water and soil is low.

PICA

The eating of earth, clay, dirt, plaster, coal, and wood has been reported from all parts of the world. Clay eating is associated with iron-deficiency anemia, and in some parts of the Middle East, is believed to be responsible for zinc deficiency in children. Absence of gastric hydrochloric acid has been shown in clay eaters in the United States and Iran. In vitro it has been demonstrated that clay can remove potassium cations from both aqueous media and serum. If this exchange also takes place in vivo, it may be responsible for iron-deficiency anemia. The cause of zinc deficiency has not been established, but preliminary laboratory investigations suggest that a similar cation-exchange mechanism may be responsible (Robson 1972).

TOXICANTS OCCURRING NATURALLY IN FOODS

Among the many chemicals which occur naturally in foods, a small number may produce undesireable effects. Substances included in this category are those which occur in foods for reasons other than as a direct result of human activity. Chiefly they are the natural components of plant and animal tissues as produced during normal growth, various other substances derived from the animal's feed or the soil or aquatic environment in which the organism grew, and compounds produced by or as a result of microbial contamination.

INTRINSIC TISSUE COMPONENTS

Of the toxicants which are intrinsic components of animal and plant tissue, the human species has in many cases evolved metabolic pathways for degrading, detoxifying, eliminating, or otherwise dealing with most, provided excessive amounts of any one are not consumed at any one time. The wider the variety of food consumed, the greater is the number of different chemical substances consumed, and the less is the chance that any one will reach a hazardous level in the diet.

Dietary oxalates consumed in high concentration can result in oxalate poisoning, and with continuous ingestion at high levels can interfere with calcium absorption and metabolism. At ordinary levels of consumption however, it is unlikely that ill effects can be observed.

Nutritional disease caused by the overconsumption of trace minerals is

TABLE 4.7
Toxicants Occurring Naturally in Food

Intrinsic Tissue Components
Oxalates
Trace minerals and metals
Lathyrogens
Solanum alkaloids
Goitrogens
Cyanogenetic glycosides
Microbial Toxins
Ergot alkaloids
Aflatoxins
Tricothecenes
Botulism

also uncommon, especially in humans who tend to consume a greater variety of foods than herbivores who are the more likely victims of mineral poisoning from naturally occurring minerals. One exception is fluoride poisoning which results from high levels of fluoride in the soil or water.

The consumption of lathyrogens is responsible for lathyrism, a crippling paralysis of the lower limbs, which is a serious health problem in certain rural areas of India, and a recurrent problem elsewhere. Lathyrism is a consequence of the excessive consumption of the seeds of the legume *Lathyrus sativus* and related species. The legume grows under adverse conditions of moisture and soil, at times when other food plants are unavailable, leaving people little choice but to depend on it. After several months, during which these seeds constitute the bulk of the diet, the paralysis gradually develops (Strong, 1976).

A steroidal alkaloid, solanidine, which occurs as a series of glycoside derivitives in market potatoes, has been responsible for some cases of human poisoning. The glycosides, collectively referred to as solanine, occurs just under the skin and particularly in the sprouts of potatoes in response to exposure to light.

Goiter is attributable mainly to iodine deficiency, but the antithyroid compounds in many plants are estimated to contribute about 4% to the world goiter incidence (Strong, 1976). Most active of these compounds are the goitrogens present in cabbage, cauliflower, brussels sprouts, broccoli, kale, kohlrabi, turnips, and rutabaga, and in the oil seed meals from rape and turnip. The antithyroid effect of goitrogens is not counteracted by dietary iodine.

Cyanogenetic glycosides occur in many plants used as human foods, in livestock feeds, and in nonfood plant products occasionally ingested, for example, by children. The most important food occurrence is that of linamarin present in cassava (manioc) and lima beans. Linamarin, like other cyanogenetic glycosides, is readily hydrolized by enzymes present in the plant tissue to release cyanide and acetone. Fatal human poisoning from cyanide rarely occurs because of the large amounts of lima bean seeds needed to provide a hazardous amount and because cassava is normally processed before use so as to reduce the cyanide concentration.

Studies of populations in West Africa, Jamaica, and Malaya consuming high levels of cassava suggest that tropical amblyopia (blindness) and tropical ataxic neuropathy, a degenerative disease, may well be caused by chronic cyanide poisoning (Strong, 1976).

MICROBIAL TOXINS

The natural food toxicants responsible for perhaps the greatest human suffering and loss of life are the mycotoxins, toxic metabolites produced by fungi which naturally infect foodstuffs.

The best known example of human poisoning by mycotoxins is "St. Anthony's Fire" caused by ergot alkaloids produced by *Claviceps purpurea* growing on cereal grain. Although a common disease in medieval times, ergotism is practically unknown today.

At present, the most widely recognized and most studied mycotoxins are the aflatoxins. Aflatoxins have been shown most probably to be responsible for Reye's syndrome in children.

The tricothecenes appear to be the mycotoxins responsible for alimentary toxic aleukia (ATA), a periodically recurring toxicosis that has killed thousands of people in Russia following the consumption of moldy grains, such as millet, in times of war and famine. Other tricothecenes produced by mold growing on rice and other grains in Japan are thought to be responsible for red mold disease of both livestock and humans.

Another important threat to human nutrition from mycotoxins arises indirectly as a result of livestock poisoning due to consumption of moldy feeds. Among other microbial toxins produced by bacteria and algae which pose a danger to humans is botulism.

DETOXIFICATION OF FOODS

Groups of people have devised methods to detoxify the foods with which they come in contact. The naturally occurring toxins in food are most commonly counteracted by cooking, and by crushing followed by extensive washing. Various chemicals may also be added, either intentionally or unintentionally, in order to detoxify foods or to increase palatability.

The cassava plant, a staple crop for a large number of tropical peoples, is easily grown, and its tuber is a reliable source of calories. There are varieties of cassava, however, which in the raw state contain glycosides which release cyanide when the plant tissues are crushed.

Cyanide, a respiratory inhibitor, is readily absorbed from the digestive tract. To detoxify the tuber, it is first rasped or grated and then soaked in water and allowed to ferment for a few days. After soaking, the shredded tuber is mashed and pressed to force out the remaining liquid, leaching out the cyanide-forming agent. The mass is then spread out to dry and the dry powder is later eaten, either dry, mixed with water to form a paste, or made into bread.

FOOD AND HUMAN SKELETAL REMAINS

By extrapolation from the material remains, and from data on contemporary or historic human populations sharing similar geographical, cultural, of technological characteristics, the patterns of a prehistoric population's diet may emerge. This information, compared with established nutrient requirements or recommendations, can be used to generate hypotheses regarding potential nutrient imbalances which may result in nutritional disorders. These hypotheses can be tested, at least in part, by examination of the human skeletal remains of an archeological population for signs of deficient or excessive nutrient intakes, and other evidence of dietary intake.

Human Skeletal Remains 5

Although examination of human skeletal remains can suggest *patterns* of nutritional disease, the limitations on the use of human skeletal material are great. The nature of nutritional diseases within a population cannot be deduced from one or two skeletons. Individuals may manifest nutritional diseases because of uniquely high nutrient requirements, disease states unrelated to dietary intakes, or malabsorption syndromes. Indications that a specific nutritional disease appears in a large proportion of the population, or in a specific at-risk group, such as women of child-bearing age, children under 5 years of age, or adults over 55 years of age, are much more important for deducing nutritional stress.

Another problem which arises in the assessment of human skeletal remains for signs of nutritional disease is that most of the signs are nonspecific, and could be attributed to a number of stresses, nutritional stress being only one possibility. Even a pattern of multiple signs can be interpreted as indicating a number of disease states. For these reasons it is important to test any hypotheses generated by the human skeletal remains against other sources of information. Does the floral, faunal, or scatalogical data support the hypothesis? Do living or historical populations, living in these circumstances, commonly display the deficiency disease suggested by the skeletal remains?

Techniques of skeletal analysis are continuously emerging and being refined. Discussion will, therefore, be limited to demographic analysis, radiographic analysis, chemical analysis, and physical examination for pathologies of nutritional origin.

DEMOGRAPHIC ANALYSIS

Mortality patterns in the first 15 years of life are sensitive to the interactions of nutritional and pathogenic elements. The greatest crisis occurs from 6 months to weaning, when the increasing nutrient demands of the infant necessitate supplementation of breast milk. When these supplementary foods are of poor nutrient quality, nutritional stress will be experienced. As supplementation increases relative to milk intake, nutritional disease may result. The supplemental period may also be accompanied by an increased incidence of severe diarrhea caused by normal intestinal biota as well as by *Shigella* and *Salmonella* organisms introduced with the new weaning foods. The frequency and duration of these diarrheal episodes increase as malnutrition becomes more severe (Scrimshaw 1966). In severe malnutrition, diarrhea may result from malabsorption of nutrients, caused by the insufficiency of proteins which form the enzymes necessary for absorption.

In such cases, disease and malnutrition are "synergistic" (Scrimshaw 1966). Each magnifies the effects of the other. Febrile disease increases metabolic rate as sepsis and trauma increase requirements for tissue repair. Gastrointestinal disease hampers nutrient absorption. Thus, disease episodes frequently precipitate kwashiorkor, scurvy, or xerophthalmia. Antibody production and tissue barriers to infection are reduced or absent in severe malnutrition, increasing the mortality rate due to childhood diseases. This is seen both in severe and in milder malnutrition states. High mortality rates in early childhood are due both to the high mortality rate associated with diarrhea, measles and other common childhood diseases, and to the frequent development of severe protein-calorie malnutrition within a few weeks of infectious episodes (Scrimshaw 1966). In either case, deaths are due to the synergism of infection and malnutrition, and would not have occurred unless both conditions were present.

The total picture is one of increased morbidity and mortality due to childhood disease. This view is supported by large-scale census data studies on the causes of infant mortality. Mortality rates in infancy show a dramatic range, accounting for most of the difference in the range of mortality from 11,621 to 1,733 post-neonatal deaths per 100,000 live births (United Nations 1955). These data are from a series of census records chosen to represent the present range of infant and adult mortality. Similarly, mortality in the 1–5-year age group is the single most variable component for age-specific deaths where life expectancy at birth varies between 22 and 74 years (Cook 1971).

A refined quantitative method of evaluating mortality curves permits measurement of mortality parameters of nutritional stress, as well as estimation of the degree to which a skeletal series deviates from the biological population it represents due to problems of preservation, recovery, and identification.

A series of models developed by a United Nations population-studies program can be used for this purpose (Cook 1971). The models can be used to demonstrate consistent patterns of over- and under-recording or mortality in several situations. The United Nations life tables are based on census data from 183 populations chosen for accuracy of recording and variety of mortality experience (United Nations 1955). Infant and early childhood mortality experiences are highly correlated with mortality experience for the population as a whole.

The models based on these tables offer applications for nutritional evaluation. They can be used up to the age of 40 for skeletal populations, that is, up to the point at which osteological evidence of age becomes increasingly less reliable. The models can be used to assess the mortality level of the population using only a subset of the age-range without taking total population size into account. If the tabulated rates for a reasonable series of models are applied to a cohort, expected deaths at the end of each period can be calculated and used to describe population mortality rates, when only a segment of the population can be studied or accurately aged. Marked deviation of the figures from reasonable populations can be taken to indicate under- or over-recording.

Demographic models have also been generated from anthropological populations, living and skeletal, historic and contemporary (Weiss 1973). The model life tables are constructed from field studies and are designed to be fit to fragmentary data. Furthermore, the models relate fertility to mortality, and allow estimation of fertility when there are no direct field data. This can be useful for nutritional analysis since not only does nutritional disease create high levels of infant mortality, but it also tends to suppress fertility through pregnancy wastage.

Using the techniques developed by Cook (1976), death rates for juveniles and adults have been examined for Late Woodland populations of the lower Illinois River region. An increased number of Late Woodland individuals in the weanling age sample, that most sensitive to the effects of malnutrition, strongly suggests that the prehistoric lifestyle during Late Woodland times was more biologically stressful than that for the earlier Middle Woodland period. Middle and Late Woodland adult mortality profiles also show directional trends. Survivorship curves indicate that the probability of survival for Middle Woodland young adults is markedly greater than that for later populations (Buikstra, 1977). These demographic shifts are associated with a suggested increase in the consumption of carbohydrates during the later Late Woodland.

Mortality profiles of archeological samples constructed to illustrate fluctuations in the relative frequencies of deaths occurring with age groups have been used to demonstrate differential physical and social stress operating at certain ages. The mortality profile of the Mississippian village site of Etowah in northwest Georgia showed that their health environment was not unlike that of the Illinois Mississippians, with the most likely ages of death including birth, the twenties, and throughout the later years. Times of relative security were during middle and late childhood and adolescence (Blakely, 1977).

CHEMICAL ANALYSIS

Human skeletal remains may be analyzed for trace elements or for carbon isotopes in an attempt to reconstruct dietary histories. Carbon isotope analysis is one of the newest techniques available for nutritional reconstructions and may be applicable to a wide variety of problems.

CARBON ISOTOPE ANALYSIS

Photosynthesis in terrestrial plants follows two main pathways: C_3, the classic Calvin pathway, and C_4, the more recently discovered Hatch-Slack pathway (Hatch and Slack 1970). During the first step of photosynthesis in the C_3 pathway, the 3-carbon molecule phosphoglyceric acid is formed, while in the C_4 pathway, the 4-carbon molecule oxaloacetate is formed. The C_3 pathway is the more widely distributed and most plants classified as browse material are C_3 plants. The C_4 pathway has a higher rate of carbon-dioxide assimilation and is an adaptation for growth in warm environments with high light intensities found mainly in tropical grasses. The two pathways can be distinguished on the basis of their respective carbon isotope ratios ($^{13}C/^{12}C$). Because C_3 plants discriminate more than do C_4 plants against the heavier isotope during uptake of atmosperic carbon-dioxide, C_3 plants consequently have a lower $^{13}C/^{12}C$ ratio than C_4 plants (Lerman and Troughton 1975).

A third group of plants depends on crassulacean acid metabolism (CAM) and can, depending on environmental conditions, fix carbon-dioxide by either the C_3 or the C_4 pathway, or both, and consequently can have C_3-like, C_4-like, or intermediate $^{13}C/^{12}C$ ratios.

The isotopic differences introduced during photosynthesis are maintained in all metabolic steps within the plant and in the subsequent animal links of the food chain of which the plants are a part. The precise ratio of these two isotopes in any given sample is measured directly (as carbon dioxide) with a mass spectrometer and the difference in parts per thousand between the ratio of the sample and that of an arbitrary carbonate standard is then calculated. The carbon isotope ratios of the collagen or carbonate fraction of bone can, in this way, provide information about the relative consumption of C_3 and C_4 plants in animal and human diets.

The $^{13}C/^{12}C$ ratios of bone from two species of hyrax has been used to distinguish a browsing species from a grazing species. The carbon isotope ratios of the bone carbonate and collagen fractions of two known species were analyzed and the carbon isotope ratios of the two diets were estimated from the bone carbon isotope ratios on the basis of controlled laboratory feeding studies.

The lower (more negative) carbon isotope ratio of the diet of the known browsers indicates that most of their diet is derived from C_3 plants, while the higher ratio of the diet of the known grazers indicates that their diet is composed largely of C_4 plants (DeNiro and Epstein 1978).

Maize is the foremost C_4 plant of economic importance, and this technique has already been applied to human and canine skeletal samples to investigate the arrival of maize in a region (Vogel and van der Marwe 1977; Burleigh and Brothwell 1978).

Information about diet can be obtained from the carbon isotope ratios of archeological bone samples if it can be shown that their original carbon isotope values have not been altered during diagenesis. The carbonate fraction of bone is usually susceptible to diagenetic alterations of its carbon isotope composition while the collagen fraction of bone is not subject to exchange with carbon in the postmortem environment and thus may preserve its original carbon isotope value. Even in cases where the collagen fraction appears to record dietary information, it must be demonstrated that changes in the concentration of collagen and its amino acid composition which may occur during diagenesis did not significantly alter its original carbon isotope ratio (DeNiro and Epstein, 1978).

Knowledge of the environmental background is needed when interpreting

TABLE 5.1

Carbon Isotope Ratios of the Diets of Two Hyrax Species Compared with Those of C_3 and C_4 Plants[a]

C_3 Plants	Browsing hyrax diet	Grazing hyrax diet	C_4 Plants
−23 to −34 per mil	−22.6 to −23.9 per mil	−12.8 to −16.0 per mil	−10 to −18 per mil

[a] Expressed as $\delta^{13}C$ values: $\delta^{13}C$ (per mil) $= \left[\dfrac{(^{13}C/^{12}C) \text{ sample}}{(^{13}C/^{12}C) \text{ standard}} -1 \right] \times 10^3$

carbon isotope data. The model situation is one in which the native plant species which may be represented in the diet, and all other cultivated plants, are C_3 plants. Marine organisms in the diet can disturb the carbon isotope ratios because they have a ^{13}C concentration close to that of C_4 plants.

TRACE ELEMENTS

A number of trace elements have been investigated in the search for reliable predictors of dietary intake (Gilbert 1975; Parker and Toots 1970). The choice of a trace element to be used for dietary reconstruction depends on its incorporation into bone from dietary sources, and its post-mortem retention in the bone mineral.

Bone mineral consists of crystals of hydroxy-apatite. Noncrystalline mineral particles may be depositied during early bone calcification followed by conversion of this noncrystalline mineral phase to crystalline apatite. The three zones of the hydroxy apatite crystal are (a) crystal interior, (b) crystal surface, and (c) hydration shell, all of which present surfaces available for the exchange of ions. The entire chemical behavior of the mineral of bone involves the transfer of ions across the hydrated crystal-solution interface. In physiological fluids, there are many ions present which are capable of substituting for calcium or phosphate in hydroxy apatite. The number of substitutions of lattice positions is limited, but at the surfaces of the crystals, the opportunities are greater. In general, it has been found that the monovalent ions of potassium, sodium, chlorine, and fluorine diffuse into the hydration shell but do not concentrate there. Multivalent anions and cations of magnesium, strontium, radium, uranium, and carbonate which are highly hydrated and/or polarizable tend to concentrate in the hydration shell, and become part of the bound-ion complex. Some of these (strontium, radium, and carbonate) enter the crystal surface itself. In addition, sodium and fluorine are known to enter the surface, and of these, strontium, radium, and fluorine can even enter the crystal interior and participate in intracrystalline exchange. The ultimate distribution of magnesium, uranium, and carbonate is not completely known, but they seem to be surface-limited. In all cases, these specific interactions involve a displacement of at least one of the normal lattice ions. Cations displace calcium, multivalent anions displace phosphate, and fluorine displaces hydroxl.

Following fossilization, two modes of occurrence of minor elements within hard tissue can be distinguished. The element can be incorporated through substitution into the apatite crystal structure, or it can occur as a separate mineral phase, filling minute voids and fractures in the bone. Of the minor elements commonly reported in fossil bone, fluorine, sodium, strontium, and yttrium are incorporated into the crystal structure, whereas silicon, manganese, and iron are restricted to the voids and fractures of the crystal (Parker and Toots 1970).

Analyses of zinc, copper, manganese, and magnesium in human hard tissue have also been performed. Zinc and copper were chosen because of their predominance in animal food, while manganese and magnesium were chosen because they occur in large amounts in vegetable foods. Results showed zinc to be a discriminator with regard to presumed animal protein whereas the remaining elements demonstrated variable results (Gilbert 1975).

Of the elements examined, strontium has become the most commonly used (Brown 1973; Gilbert 1975; Schoeninger 1979; Szpunar 1977). Strontium is incorporated into bone in the same manner as calcium, but systematically discriminated against in favor of calcium during the process of bone deposition. Since the body also preferentially excretes strontium, as little as one-eighth as much ingested strontium as compared to ingested calcium is incorporated into bone (Kulp, Eckelmann, and Schulert 1957).

Plants absorb strontium from the soil along with the necessary calcium. There appears to be little discrimination against strontium in favor of calcium by plants (Comar, Russell, and Wasserman 1957). Continued movement of strontium from soil through plant stems into the leaves and storage organs results in higher concentrations of strontium in the leaves and in storage than in stems. In addition, succulent herbaceous vegetation (shrubs) accumulate higher strontium concentrations than do grasses. On the basis of this differential accumulation, vertebrate browsers have been distinguished from grazers (Toots and Voorhies 1965).

The amount of strontium deposited in the bony parts of animals depends on the rate of strontium passage through biological membranes, and on the amount of the element available to the animal. Strontium becomes concentrated in the flesh of marine and freshwater molluscs and crustaceans, and marine vertebrates have higher levels of strontium in their skeleton than do terrestrial vertebrates (Kulebakina, 1975; Odum, 1957; Ophel, 1963; Rosenthal, 1963; Schroeder, Tipton, and Nason 1972).

Terrestrial vertebrates incorporate strontium in their skeletons in direct proportion to the amount of strontium in their diet. Since strontium is discriminated against in the process of absorption and deposition, the tissues of herbivores will contain less strontium than the plants which form their diet. Strontium is further discriminated against before deposition into the tissues of carnivores who initially consume less strontium than the herbivores which form the carnivores' diet. Omnivores, consuming both plants and animals, can be expected to display intermediate strontium tissue levels.

Studies on bone strontium levels between bones of an individual indicate that there is no difference other than that expected from measurement error

TABLE 5.2
Sr/Ca Ratios in Plants, Carnivores, and Herbivores

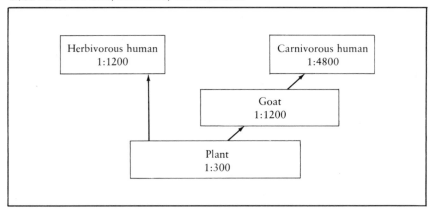

(Hodges *et al.* 1950; Thurber, Kulp, Hodges, Gast, and Wampler 1958; Wessen, Ruddy, Gustafson, and Irwin 1977; Yablonskii 1971, 1973). The evidence is inconclusive for age-dependent differences in strontium incorporation. Because of the differences of opinion, a consideration of the ages of the individuals within the sample must be made and reported.

Control for natural differences in the strontium content of soil and water can be achieved if comparisons are based on material from a single fossil quarry, since strontium levels in the soil vary with proximity to large bodies of water, with the salinity of the soil, leaching of the soil, and the principle mineral of the soil. Homogeneous samples of fossil biotic communities are prerequisites for meaningful analysis (Toots and Voorhies 1965).

Techniques for strontium analysis are varied, but most rely on flame emission or atomic absorption spectroscopy, although neutron activation has also been used. Most also agree on the need for ultrasonic cleaning to avoid soil contamination (Brown 1974; Brown and Keyzer 1978; Schoeninger 1979; Szpunar, Lambert, and Buikstra 1978).

The ability to reconstruct food chains using strontium analysis can be applied to a variety of dietary problems. The changes in diet through time at a specific site can be documented through changes in bone strontium levels. The relative importance of meat in comparison to vegetable food in the diet at any one point in time can be approached by the comparison of human-bone strontium levels to those of known carnivores, herbivores, and omnivores from the same site. Lastly, differences between subgroups within a population can also be identified. Such dietary differences, which result from differential access to meat, may occur between status levels, between males and females, between young and old, or between occupational groups.

RADIOGRAPHIC ANALYSIS

Two markers of growth arrest, suggestive of malnutrition, have been discovered by radiographic analysis: metacarpal notches and transverse lines of increased density, which are also referred to as Harris lines.

METACARPAL NOTCHING

Metacarpal notches were reported in approximately 72% of a longitudinal sample of Alabama children undergoing mild nutritional stress (Dreizen, Snodgrass, Webb-Peploe, and Spiess 1958; Dreizen, Sparks, and Stine 1965). The notches appear in the proximal metacarpals and in distal metacarpal I at some time during development. This lesion is more frequent in males than in females, perhaps supporting the theory that males are more sensitive to environmental trauma during their development. The lesion is also more extensive in slow-growing than in fast-growing children. The notches apparently arise from the irregular fusion of pseudo-epiphyses. They are obliterated by age 13 in females and 15 in males. Although data on the environmental variables related to this marker are scanty, and the age range of incidence is narrow, investigation in skeletal series might be useful, since such notches could be observable in skeletal populations recovered from archaeological sites.

The occurrence of notching in normal Ohio children is 100%, although some of the notching is very light (Lee and Garn 1967). The high incidence of metacarpal notching described in the Alabama sample may be attributable to the greater percentage of more marked notching, which is occasioned by the slowing down of the growth process. In Ohio boys, a trend was observed in differences in stature between markedly notched and less markedly notched groups. Less markedly notched groups were taller than the more markedly notched groups. This trend however was not observed in females (Lee, Garn and Rohmann 1968).

TRANSVERSE LINES OF INCREASED DENSITY

The lines and bands which may appear on the tibia and fibula upon radiographic examination, as well as on the calcaneus, the epiphyses, the ileum and the ischium, or on the scapula, are radiographically visible because of increased mineral density (Garn, Silverman, Hertzog, and Rohmann 1968). The lines are associated with episodes of disease in childhood and possibly adolescence. Increased density, however, may also result from the presence of lead, bismuth, or other heavy metals, dense bone formation, small trabeculae with thick walls, or all three together (Garn and Baby 1969).

New lines can be shown following a large number of therapeutic situations; transfusions in treatment of chronic and acute anemia, testosterone therapy for pituitary growth failure, administration of human growth hormone, and rehabilitation of patients with protein-calorie malnutrition. Lines and bands can also be related to hypervitaminosis D, to lead poisoning as a result of pica (ingestion of nonfood items), and to phosphorus poisoning in infancy and childhood. Even prenatal events may be represented, as may be adjustment to the extrauterine environment (Garn et al. 1968).

The mechanism by which transverse lines form has been demonstrated in rats by experimental dietary restriction (Park 1954, 1964; Park and Richter 1953). Dietary restriction results in the deposition of only a thin transverse bone stratum which is termed the primary stratum. This is formed by the continued osteoblastic activity after epiphyseal cartilage growth has stopped. When normal nutrition resumes, the cartilage cells recover in 4–9 days, and are ready for invasion from the osteoblasts. The osteoblasts, however, recover immediately and, over the primary stratum, lay down a thick transverse secondary stratum which is termed the recovery factor. Transverse lines, therefore, are not lines of arrested growth, but recovery lines representing periods of renewed growth after growth arrest. Starvation alone is not sufficient for transverse line formation, but must be *followed* by adequate nutrition. Therefore a population subjected to chronic malnutrition may not display as many lines as a population experiencing periods of acute malnutrition followed by periods of adequate nutrition.

Typically, new lines appear after the first year (Schwager 1968). The number of new lines peaks in the second or third year and diminishes after the fifth year. New lines rarely appear in adolescence. This agrees with the nutritional data which show that nutritional stress typically begins during weaning and continues to be most important during the first 5 years of life. New transverse lines on the distal tibia are more common among males than females. This is consistent with the theory that males are more vulnerable to environmental trauma during the growth period. Alternatively, it may reflect a greater rate of subperiosteal apposition and linear growth of bone in males. The lines however do not persist as long in males as in females, perhaps due to enhanced bone remodeling in males. Females, therefore, show fewer lines on the average, but there is a greater prevalence of persisting transverse lines on the distal tibia in females (Schwager 1968).

The distance between a pair of transverse lines on both the proximal and distal ends of the tibia remain stable over time. The majority of lines appear on both the right and left limbs, exhibiting bilateral symmetry (Garn and Baby 1968). On the basis of longitudinal radiographic data for children subject to regular and periodic medical examination, a clear-cut statistically significant, but low-order, association was found to exist between illness or trauma, and the appearance of a new line on the distal tibia (Garn et al. 1968).

In prehistoric California populations, the average number of transverse lines in the distal femur is 8, although in modern North American adults, transverse lines are much less frequently observed. In Ohio adults, only 25% of 160 women and 12% of 86 men had any lines extending at least halfway across the distal tibia. The age of death somewhat correlates with the frequency of lines in the prehistoric California sample. In that sample, individuals who died between the ages of 18 and 30 had an average of 8.5 lines, whereas those who survived past 30 had an average of 6.9 lines. Males and females in the sample had nearly identical frequencies of transverse lines (McHenry 1968). The greater frequency of transverse lines in those who died between 18 and 30 may suggest the better health of those with fewer lines who lived to be older than 30. On the other hand, what is seen may merely reflect the inclusion in the group over 30 of those over 50 who have lost transverse lines due to age-associated subperiosteal apposition and endosteal surface absorption, which reach a maximum rate between the 50th and 60th year and continue through the later years.

PALEOPATHOLOGIES OF THE BONES

Of the nutritional diseases which create skeletal pathologies, the most frequently encountered are rickets and its adult counterpart, osteomalacia, as well as hypervitaminosis D, scurvy, and hypervitaminosis and hypovitaminosis A. Chronic malnutrition, which is reflected in reduced adult stature, and iron-deficiency anemia, are less commonly identified.

RICKETS AND OSTEOMALACIA

Rickets and its counterpart found in adults, osteomalacia, are defined arbitrarily as a bone or skeleton containing too much osteoid (unmineralized bone matrix) compared to a suitable standard of normal. Although the diseases are generally attributed to vitamin D deficiency, there are many types of osteomalacia which may vary according to their various dynamic and chemical characteristics (Frost 1964).

Normally, the amount of new osteoid produced is the same as the amount of new bone produced. In a steady state, the amount of osteoid converted to bone is equal to the amount of osteoid formed. The existence of osteomalacia means that these two processes of matrix formation and mineralization are out of balance so that an accumulation of osteoid could occur (Frost 1964).

The main cause of nutritional rickets and osteomalacia is an insufficiency of vitamin D, which may be due to inadequate dietary intake or lack of sufficient exposure to sunlight. In the absence of an adequate amount of vitamin D, there is a reduction in the absorption of calcium and, apparently, also of phosphorus from the intestinal tract, making less available to the skeleton. As a result, the deposition of bone mineral is diminished. The resorption of calcium from ossified bone and its replacement by osteoid makes the bones both pliable and fragile, and hence susceptible to distortions, curvatures, and fractures (Jaffee 1972).

The characteristic features of rickets resulting from vitamin D deficiency are (a) general retardation of skeletal growth; (b) development of frontal and parietal bossing; (c) light and brittle bone texture; (d) abnormally high arching of the temporal bone; (e) forward curvature of the femur, an exaggeration of the slight normal curve of this bone; (f) curvature of the tibia, fibula, ulna, and radius; (g) development of knock-knees or bow-legs; and (h) asymmetry and distortion of the chest resulting from a slight lateral curvature of the spine (scoliosis) (Dick 1922).

In rachitic infants, the only manifestation may be some widening of the calcarial sutures and the anterior fontenal. At 6–9 months the frontal region may show some bossing, and the anterior fontenal will be large. The head of the rachitic infant is likely to show some deformation from flattening on one side or in the back. Beading of the costochondral junctions may be prominent. The thoracic cage may appear further deformed from exaggerated forward protrusion of the sternum and from a flaring of the costal margin along the attachment of the diaphragm. In addition, enlargement at the wrist and ankle may be prominent, and there may even be the beginnings of curvature of the long bones. By 2 years of age, the rachitic child displays exaggerations of the earlier signs. Because of the increased prominence of parietal bossing, together with depression of the anterior fontenal and coronal and sagittal sutures, the top of the head may appear flat and squarish. Delay in dental eruption may be present (Jaffee 1972). In those teeth which have erupted, the enamel may be defective near the gums.

In the thoracic cage of the young child, exaggeration of skeletal change is shown by increased protrusion of the sternum and indentation of the chest wall along the lines of the costochondral junction. There may also be some dorsal curvature of the spine. The enlargement of the ends of the long bones at the wrists and ankles increases in prominence, and enlargement is also shown by the bone ends at the knees and elbows. The proximal and middle phalanges of the fingers may be thickened and the joints between them may appear constricted.

In adults, thickening of the vault of the skull may be observed, although not in every case. When present, it is not found evenly distributed over the vault but usually affects the frontal and parietal bones. The top of the head in advanced rickets is marked by prominent frontal and parietal bossing (Jaffee 1972).

Changes at the costochondral junctions in advanced cases initiate the deformation of the thoracic cage. The deformity may consist merely of a furrow at each side of the sternum caused by sinking in of the ribs in the region of the junction. The body of the sternum may have been pushed forward, the manubrium elevated, and the xyphoid pointed inward. The clavicles may show increased anterior bowing. Muscle weakness favors the development of dorsal kyphosis. If the bones of the pelvis and those of the lower extremities also become distorted, the thorax may become further altered through the development of a scoliosis and a lumbar lordosis.

In some cases, the epiphyseal–diaphyseal junctions of the long bones may be enlarged. In some of the bones, the epiphysis and the rachitic intermediate zone may be tilted upon the diaphysis. Curvature of the bone shaft results from the misdirection of growth, but may also arise from fracture. On the whole, the long bones of upper extremities are less likely to show severe curvatures than those of the lower extremities which support the weight of the body. The shaft of the humerus may bow outward, while the radius and the ulna may show exaggerations of their normal curvature. In the lower extremities, the most typical deformities encountered are bow-legs and knock-knees. The deformity of the lower vertebral column contributes to the pelvic deformity characteristic of the disease (Jaffee 1972).

HYPERVITAMINOSIS D

In both children and adults, intoxication from hypervitaminosis D produces a number of skeletal signs. Young children who have received large doses of vitamin D reveal the presence of narrow bands of radiopacity at sites of endochondral bone growth. The increased density of the bands reflects the heavy calcification of the matrix of the proliferating cartilage. Further along the bone shafts, the metaphyses may appear less opaque because of the presence of focal osteoporosis. Vitamin D intoxication may also be the basis for metastatic calcification involving blood vessels, various organs, and para-articular tissues.

In hypervitaminosis D, the bones of adults show evidence of osteoporosis. Calcifications form through the deposition of calcium in bursae neighboring upon joints, or overlying bony prominences, in tendon sheaths, and sometimes even within articular capsules. In addition to mediating the absorption of calcium, vitamin D can also mobilize mineral bone to elevate serum calcium levels, and it is this elevated serum calcium level which results in the calcifications (McLean and Urist 1961).

SCURVY

In general, scurvy is characterized by a hemorrhagic tendency which results from vitamin C deficiency. Not only is subperiosteal hemorrhage involved, but also changes at various sites of endochondral bone formation (Jaffee 1972). The latter changes are most striking at the costochondral junction of the ribs and at the epiphyseal–diaphyseal junctions of the long bones, that is, at sites where endochondral bone formation is most active. When advanced, the alterations induced by scurvy at these sites include the occurrence of infractions and fractures on the shaft side.

The ribs in affected children present sharp, firm ridges at the cartilage–shaft junction, and subperiosteal hemorrhage occurs along the shaft. Junctional beading results from subperiosteal hemorrhage and from depression and displacement of the cartilage backward and inward in consequence of infraction or fracture of the rib shaft near the junction. Adolescents and young adults display junctional changes in addition to subperiosteal hemorrhage (Jaffee 1972). In advanced scurvy, the long bones show hemorrhagic effusion under the periosteum. In affected bone, the effusion may have elevated the periosteum at one or both ends or even over its entire length.

These characteristics are the consequence of failure of formation and maintenance of intercellular material. All intercellular substances of supporting tissues—bone cartilage, fibrous connective tissue, and dentin—have in common a matrix largely made up of collagen, and this material in scurvy either is not produced, or produced in defective form.

Microscopic examination of a costochondral junction shows that the cartilage cells at the proliferation zone are not regularly arranged. Extending shaftward for some distance from the proliferation zone, is observed a lattice-work of trabeculae of calcified cartilage matrix, free of borders of osseous tissue. Throughout the junctional region, there is extensive resorption of whatever cortical and spongy bone was present in the junctional area before the onset of scurvy (Jaffee 1972).

Scorbutic bone lesions result from cessation of matrix deposition and the formation of reticular cells by the osteoblasts. The mechanism of calcification is not affected, but abnormal connective tissue formed during vitamin C deficiency is not calcifiable. The effects of the deficiency are reversible (McLean and Urist 1961). This picture is produced mainly as osteoblastic activity is depressed and, consequently, wherever osseous tissue would normally be forming, the deposition of collagenous bone matrix by the osteoblasts is reduced or arrested (Jaffee 1972).

HYPOVITAMINOSIS AND HYPERVITAMINOSIS A

Vitamin A is essential for activities of epiphyseal cartilage cells, whose failure results in supression of endochondral growth of bone. Remodeling sequences also cease to operate, although appositional growth of periosteal origin continues. These effects lead to abnormalities in the shapes of bones and the failure of certain bony foramina to enlarge, bringing pressure on various nerves (McLean and Urist 1961).

In relation to vitamin A intoxication, although there have been observed clinical instances of hypervitaminosis A in both children and adults, the skeletal manifestations of vitamin A intoxication have been noted only in older infants and very young children. The ingestion of large amounts of vitamin A over a long period of time may certainly lead to the development of cortical hyperstosis. Occasionally hypervitaminosis A may also be found to adversely affect the epiphyseal cartilage plates in affected children. In some cases, retardation of the longitudinal growth of bones, due to damaging effects upon their epiphyseal cartilage plates, has been noted. Also, broadening of the shafts of the lower ends of the femur and upper end of the tibia may result from disordered local remodeling (Jaffee 1972).

Hypervitaminosis A may also lead to fragility and subsequent fractures of the long bones. Under the influence of excessive vitamin A, acid hydrolases are released from lysosomes and their proteolytic activity results in the breakdown of the protein component of the protein polysaccharide of the matrix.

PROTEIN-CALORIE MALNUTRITION

When insufficient calories and protein are available during childhood and adolescence, growth is suppressed to conserve calories needed to maintain basic body processes. If calories and protein become available before adulthood, growth may resume, and the individual may regain a normal height. In situations however where malnutrition is chronic, adult stature will be less than that for well-nourished individuals.

When fairly complete skeletal populations can be recovered from archeological sites, stature estimation is possible using published tables and formulas based on individuals whose stature during life was known (Trotter and Gleser 1958). Lower limb bones generally furnish a better measure of stature than do those of the upper limbs. The best correlation is between stature and the sum of the femoral and fibular lengths. For Mesoamerican skeletal samples, another set of tables and formulas have been published, derived from a sample of Mexican cadavers (Genoves 1967). Many investigators use these formulas for all prehistoric New World skeletal populations.

Stature estimation can be used to examine long-term changes in resource availability and nutritional intakes, and to test the possibility of status differences within a population. It has been suggested (Haviland 1967) that at Tikal taller stature associated with high social status (as indicated by burial in tombs) was due to dietary as well as genetic factors (Haviland 1967).

From published Mexican archaeological samples for four sites (Nickens, 1976), a decline in male stature has been noted over time, and is suggested to be an adaptation to the consequences of food production.

IRON-DEFICIENCY ANEMIA

Iron-deficiency anemia is less commonly a result of inadequate dietary iron than of poor absorption or heavy iron losses. Poor iron absorption is associated with protein-poor diets, and heavy iron losses are frequently the result of hemorrhage and parasitic infection, including malaria. The changes produced by chronic iron-deficiency anemia are nonspecific and may also be the result of chronic infection, trauma, or possibly other diseases. Finding signs of iron-deficiency anemia can only suggest that the disease was present, and other evidence should be sought. A series of cranial lesions, generally lumped together under the term symmetrical osteoporosis, which includes osteoporotic pitting, cribra orbitalia, and porotic hyperstosis, are generally indicative of iron-deficiency anemia. Radiographic examination usually reveals a hair-on-end pattern of the bone mineral. Cribra orbitalia has been demonstrated to be the result of iron-deficiency anemia in early Nubian populations (Carlson *et al.* 1974).

PALEOPATHOLOGY OF THE DENTITION

Although dental pathologies tend to be nonspecific and cannot generally indicate a particular nutritional disease, their presence is often used to suggest nutritional stress. An exception to the lack of specificity is the nutritional disease fluorosis. Fluorosis, or fluoride poisoning, is the result of excessive fluoride intake, usually from natural sources in the water or from food grown in soil containing high fluoride levels. In early stages the teeth display white flecks in the enamel. In later stages of the disease, the teeth become stained with a brown pigment. In the advanced stages the teeth are pitted and have a corroded appearance.

ENAMEL HYPOPLASIA AND DENTAL ASYMMETRY

Enamel hypoplasia and dental asymmetry have been used as indicators of generalized nutritional and health stress. Dental enamel hypoplasia, a developmental arrest of enamel during the process of crown formation, is attributed to occurrences of malnutrition and other disease processes during childhood. Adverse or stressful environmental conditions during growth may also disturb the natural bilateral symmetry of the dentition. In living human populations dental asymmetry is greatest among those whose health, nutritional, and general socioeconomic status is lowest (Perzigian, 1977). To express the magnitude of metric asymmetry, correlation coefficients (r) between pairs of antimeric teeth are used. The proportion of intraindividual variation due to asymmetry is equal to 1-r. This difference estimates the amount of variation due to nongenetic, environmental factors that have deflected an organism off its course toward bilateral symmetry. A high level of dental asymmetry at the Indian Knoll site, a Late Archaic site in west central Kentucky, is associated with a number of other indicators of nutritional stress. In addition, within the Indian Knoll population, the taller individuals have less asymmetrical teeth than shorter individuals (Perzigian, 1977).

DENTAL CARIES AND PERIDONTAL DISEASE

Dental caries and peridontal disease have been attributed to nutritional stress, high carbohydrate diets, and vitamin C deficiency. Nutritional stress results in defective tooth structure which is more susceptible to disease while a high carbohydrate diet promotes the formation of dental plaque which is associated with both dental caries and peridontal disease. Vitamin C deficiency weakens the structure surrounding the teeth, leading to peridontal disease.

Dental caries can result from a variety of carious lesions. In enamel caries, the enamel itself is invaded and destroyed by bacteria; while at other times cementum (the outer covering of the root of the tooth) and dentine may become necrotic, and the necrotic material is invaded by bacteria. The latter process resembles the infection of necrotic areas elsewhere in the body and differs only in that the teeth tend to be more vulnerable (Little 1973).

Well-formed teeth, with an adequate supply of vitamin D present during their formation are less susceptible to enamel caries than poorly formed teeth. An adequate supply of fluoride is also required during the time of tooth formation. Lesions spread from defects in the surface; thus, the better formed the tooth, the fewer the defects.

The destructive agents that can penetrate through these weak points are acids and bacteria. The organic component is attacked first, and it is the less dense protein that is vulnerable. The crystallites are as likely to be washed away as to be dissolved away. Starches as well as sugars are involved, since starches may contain proteolytic compounds which would help to initiate the lesion. Such a lesion would be expected to advance slowly.

Teeth susceptible to the characteristic and fairly rapidly developing lesions have protein in a less chemically stable form than normal, which would facilitate the spread of these lesions. Circumstantial evidence indicates that the incidence of dental caries is affected by the degree of stress, nutritional as well, to which the individual is subjected. The most important effect of stress on enamel caries is a rise in the level of excess cortisol in the blood. This cortisol stimulates connective tissue to produce proteolytic enzymes. There is also a physiological rise in pregnancy, and often a series of temporary rises in cortisol level during adolescence. The assumption is that enzymes diffusing from odontoblasts in a phagocytic phase have partly degraded protein in the neighboring enamel (Little 1973).

Poor diet, then, is implicated in at least three stages of lesion formation: (a) in the formation of defective enamel and protein which is more susceptible to bacterial invasion; (b) in the introduction of proteolytic compounds which attack the protein; and (c) in the creation of stress which increases cortisol levels.

The consumption of high levels of dietary carbohydrates has been linked to the accumulation of dental plaque which may be responsible for dental caries and peridontal disease. The metabolic activity of dental plaque is mainly due to its microbial content which exists in an extrabacterial matrix.

Dietary carbohydrates are of primary importance in leading to the colonization of microorganisms on tooth surfaces and permitting plaque microorganisms to sustain their life functions even under periods of nutritional stress.

Dietary carbohydrate contributes to the disease potential of oral microorganisms through its role in the formation of dental plaque and through supporting the metabolic activity of plaque microflora which yield bacterial products that directly interact with oral hard and soft tissue or elicit a host response.

Since dental plaque is an essentially anaerobic environment, the utilization of exogenous carbohydrates must be done by fermentation. Fermentation products, generally acidic in nature, have the potential to damage oral tissue. Lactic acid, the fermentation product most universally produced, is generally considered to be the major contributor to the acidic pH of dental plaque and is thought to play a major role in the etiology of oral disease by participating in the demineralization of enamel and cementum in coronal and root surface caries (Brown, 1976).

Other products of oral microorganisms have been implicated as having a role in the creation of dental caries and peridontal disease. Their biosynthesis at levels sufficient to damage oral tissues or elicit a host response is generally dependent on the production of energy from carbohydrate fermentation. These products include a number of enzymes which collectively have the potential to degrade the organic components of enamel and dentin, disrupt the intercellular matrix of the oral epithelium, destroy connective tissue components, alter cell surfaces and cellular permeability, disrupt cell-cell adhesion, and initiate an acute inflammatory response (Brown, 1976).

DENTAL ATTRITION

Dental attrition is associated with the ingestion of food containing abrasive material, and with many nonmasticatory functions. A rapid rate of tooth attrition will prompt morphological changes in the tooth itself, especially in the root area, with pronounced deposition of secondary cementum on the root surfaces, and withdrawal of the neural and nutritional supply to the tooth.

The degree and type of wear differ between populations practicing various dietary strategies. This variation in wear reflects differences in diet, food preparation techniques, tool use, and sexual division of labor (Molnar, 1971, 1972). Whether through mastication of food, chewing hides, or cracking open shells, attrition reflects the contact of people with their environment and can serve as a source of information on diet.

CONCLUSION

The estimation of human nutrient requirements and the examination of the human skeletal remains can be used to generate hypotheses which one can test by the study of the floral, faunal, and material remains. In order to propose meaningful hypotheses, it is essential that the physiological processes which create nutrient requirements, and which affect the human skeleton, be understood. Study of the human skeletal remains for the purpose of dietary reconstruction is inadequate by itself. The evidence provided by the human skeleton is, for the most part, general in nature and can suggest a number of possibilities from which one chooses on the basis of evidence obtained from the floral, faunal, and material remains.

Archeological Remains Related to Subsistence 6

Material culture is the substance of archeology and the basis on which past ways of life are reconstructed. It is not the intention to give a complete review of this subject here but merely to point out some of the implications of the diverse array of archeological remains to subsistence. The vagaries of perservation have resulted in unequal representation of different subsistence activities. Generally, little evidence remains to document tubers gathered in a basket and brought back to the site for a meal. On the other hand, deer bones and flint spear points preserved in a site may attest to prehistoric hunting. The basic tool kit of the primary subsistence activities, gathering, fishing, hunting, agriculture, and food processing, will be discussed and some of the diverse lines of evidence relating to these activities will be reviewed.

GATHERING

Gathering is a subsistence activity that has great antiquity and importance to the prehistoric diet. Gathered resources have probably accounted for a major portion of the prehistoric diet, particularly in the region between the middle latitudes (39°N and 39°S) (Murdock 1967). It is also an activity that was engaged in primarily by women. Despite the importance of this activity to subsistence, equipment used in gathering is rarely preserved.

A distinction must be made between foraging, in which each individual goes out and eats what is collected on the spot, and gathering, in which food is collected and brought back to camp to share with members of the family. The most dramatic evidences of gathering are the huge shell middens, found in many coastal regions as well as along the courses of some rivers. It is most likely that a container of some sort, a modified gourd, basket, box, or bag made of woven, matted, or netted fabric, or animal skin, was used to carry the gathered molluscs from the oyster bars or clam beds to the occupation site that became a shell midden. Clearly many other gathered resources, such as nuts and berries, could be brought back to the occupation site most efficiently in a container.

When viewed from the standpoint of net energy, gathering is prohibitively costly without the use of a container which makes it possible to reduce the number of trips between the food source and the home. Many animals that gather food for subsequent storage or sharing have "solved" the problem of a container by anatomical means. Ground squirrels can carry large quantities of food in their cheek pouches. Pocket gophers have external pockets that they can also fill with food. Human beings, of course, have satisfied the need for a container in many cultural ways (Figure 6.1).

The techniques and materials used in the construction of containers such as baskets are exceedingly varied. The materials from which baskets or fabrics are made are plant or animal fibers. Suitable fiber is found almost everywhere. Many different techniques have been developed to use different materials in different methods of basket and fabric construction. The plant and animal materials are all perishable and subject to decay. Therefore

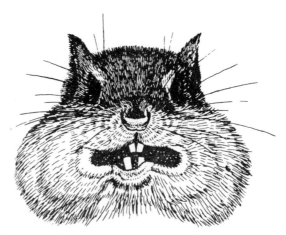

Figure 6-1. An eastern chipmunk with his pouches full, having "solved" the need for a bag for efficient gathering (reprinted by permission of Louisiana State University Press from *The Mammals of Louisiana and its adjacent waters* by George H. Lowery 1974:197).

remnants are preserved in only a few areas, such as the dry interiors of caves where the changes of the climate cannot penetrate. Examples of basketry are, however, known from the Mesolithic, and this technology probably extends back into the Late Paleolithic (Spier 1970).

FISHING

Netting, one technique of fabric construction, has many uses, one of which is fishing. As with other fabrics, netting is made of a variety of fibers, all of which are perishable. One type of netting construction, a seine, may have weights on one side and floats on the other so that when pulled through the water it maintains its vertical position for greatest efficiency in recovering fish. The netting and floats are made of perishable plant fibers and other plant parts. The weights are usually stone or shell that have been grooved or pierced so thay can be securely tied to the edge of the netting. Stone weights can also be wrapped, in the same way bolo stones are wrapped, and the wrapping tied to the netting (Cumbaa, personal communication). Upon deterioration of the wrapping, these weights would be difficult'to recognize. Only the regular position of a row of weights might give a clue to the former existence of a seine (Figure 6.2).

Netting supported by a hoop or triangle of rigid material, such as a woody vine or rod, has also been put to wide use. The matayagual, netting approximately a meter in diameter suspended from a wooden hoop, is still used in parts of the gulf coast of Mexico (Figure 6.3). It almost certainly has great antiquity, although archeological remains of these nets have not been recovered. Their construction and design are dictated by tradition and follow a precise pattern.

Some types of equipment are designed for capture of only one kind of prey, whereas other equipment may have more general use. The matayagual, as it is used in Mexico today, is most general. When children are not using it to catch each other or grasshoppers and dragonflies, it is used to catch small birds or lizards. Its main use, however, is to gather the small fishes, crayfishes, and molluscs that live along the water's edge.

In the absence of actual netting remains, the use of netting may also be inferred from the types of fishes recovered in the site. The recovery of remains of schooling, herbivorous fishes, particularly small ones, strongly suggests that netting of some sort was used to catch this resource.

Carnivorous fishes may be caught with nets as well as with the use of other types of equipment, such as hooks, gorges, and traps, that takes advantage of their carnivorous feeding behavior. As with netting, hooks and traps are made in different ways using various materials. The simplest type

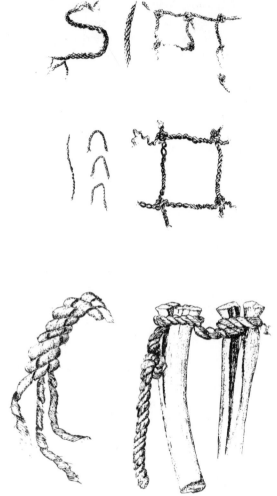

Figure 6-2. Netting found in archeological context from the Key Marco site, southwest coast of Florida. These specimens clearly show the way the cord was made, the kind of knot that was tied, and the attachment of the wooden peg floats (reprinted by permission of the University Presses of Florida from *The Material culture of Key Marco Florida* by Marian S. Gilliland 1975:figs. 4 and 5).

of hook is the gorge, a slender pointed sliver of bone or spine tied in the middle with a line. It functions by lodging in the fishes' throat, and, when caught, the fish can be pulled in. Hooks may be simple, in the shape of a semicircle or oval with an attachment for a line on one side and often with a barb on the other side of the curve (Figure 6.4). These hooks are made of such materials as bone, shell, coconut shell, turtle shell, or even of gold. Hooks may be compound, composed of several elements bound together. A single element of a compound hook may be difficult to recognize in an archeological context, when it is found separate from its formerly associated parts.

Traps may be active, luring a fish into an enclosure from which it cannot escape, or passive, relying on the behavior of the fish. The baited trap may be in the form of a barrel or box with a funnel-like entrance. Such traps are usually made of perishable materials. Their use may escape casual notice as they would be underwater, and their location might be kept secret from other members of the community.

The filtering action of a trap may be reflected in the fish remains recovered in a site. The size of the entrance to the trap will eliminate individuals too large to pass freely into the trap, and the spaces in the fabric of the trap will allow small fishes to escape. What will be found are fishes that conform closely to one size. Wiers or tidal traps are often situated in estuaries, where, during high tide, the fish may swim freely in and out, but become stranded as the tide recedes. Wiers may be made of wooden pilings or stone walls. The less perishable stone walls may persist as prominent features for a long time. The same principals are used in constructing traps to catch terrestrial animals, that is, the animals may be funneled into a coral or trap and their escape prevented by blocking the entrance.

Spears are another major tool category used for fishing as well as hunting. Spears are modified in a number of ways for catching various kinds of

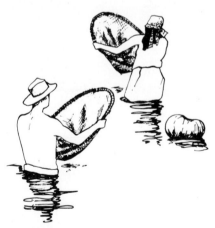

Figure 6-3. Two people using a dip net called a Matayagual to catch small fish and crayfish along the banks of an oxbow lake from the Rio Coatzacoalcos, Vera Cruz, Mexico. The catch is put in the gourd that floats beside them. (drawn from a photograph by Lynn C. Balck)

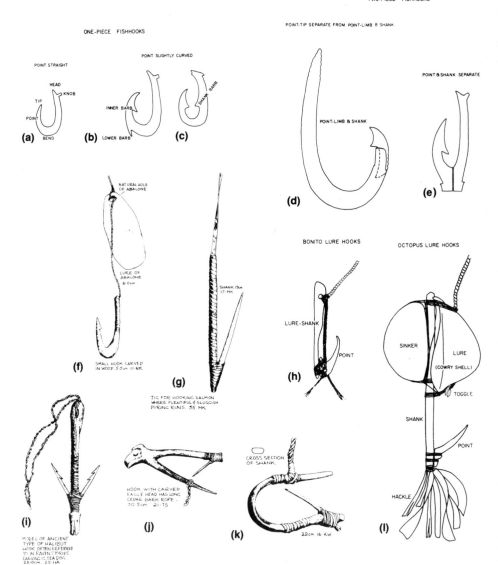

Figure 6-4. Hooks may be simple or compound and are made in different ways and of a great variety of materials. Examples from Hawaii (a, b, c, d, e, h, i) and the northwest coast (f, g, j, k, l). (Reprinted by permission of the Bishop Museum Press from *Hawaiian archaeology fishhooks* by K. P. Emory, W. J. Bonk, and Y. H. Simoto 1968:8, 9, 11 and of Douglas and McIntyre from *Indian Fishing: Early methods on the Northwest coast* by Hilary Stewart 1977:37, 43, 50)

fishes, aquatic mammals, and reptiles. Different categories of fishing spears are distinguished by the number of different points combined on the shaft and whether the point is detachable. A simple spear has a shaft with a fixed point that sometimes has barbs. A spear shaft with two or more barbed or unbarbed points shafted to it is called a leister. A harpoon is a type of spear with a removable point which is usually tied to the spear shaft or a float. The shafts of most of these types of spears are wood, and the points are usually made of wood or bone.

HUNTING

Spears used for killing terrestrial animals are usually simple, with a fixed point, but may be propelled in different ways. Spears may simply be hurled at the prey. However, use of a spear thrower (an atlatl) multiplies the effectiveness of the spear by greatly increasing the velocity of the spear. This greater speed, which increases the range of the weapon as well as its penetration power, is gained by the mechanical advantage afforded by the spear thrower which in effect lengthens the hunter's arm (Figure 6.5). The effectiveness of a short spear (or arrow) is still further increased when propelled by a bow.

Rarely do we find the "smoking pistol," although finds of the skeletal remains of animals with a projectile point lodged in a vital spot have been reported (Cumbaa 1972; Noe-Nygaard 1975) (Figure 6.6). A convincing case has also been made for a hunting technique based on healed and unhealed bone injuries in prey species (Noe-Nygaard 1975). Repeated finds

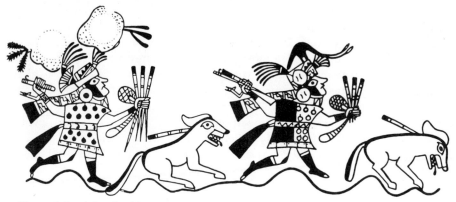

Figure 6-5. A fine line Mochica drawing of a hunting scene. The hunters are using spear throwers (reprinted from *Moche art and iconography* by permission of the author Christopher B. Donnan 1976:135).

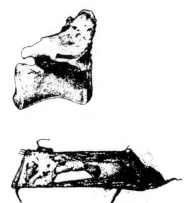

Figure 6-6. Projectile points lodged in the lumbar vertebra of a red deer (*Cervus elaphus*). Top shows the vertebra with the unhealed fracture. Bottom shows an enlargement of the fracture with the wedged flint fragments probably derived from an arrow point (reprinted by permission of North-Holland Press and the author from *Bone injuries caused by human weapons* by Nanna Noe-Nygaard 1975:158).

of piercing injuries to the scapulae of red deer (*Cervus elaphus*) and skulls of pigs (*Sus scrofa*) are interpreted as injuries caused by the hunter's spear thrust and penetration of the animal's vital spots (Figure 6.7).

Graphic representations can provide a rare glimpse of a tool in use. The superb realistic art of the Mochicas, created around the time of Christ on the coast of Peru, gives detailed insight into many aspects of Mochica life. Use of the atlatl is clearly illustrated in the fine-line drawing of the fox hunt (Figure 6.5). Equally graphic is the use of a net in hunting deer (Figure 6.8).

Artistic representations, such as petroglyphs, three dimensional carved or modelled statues, or painted figures, may reveal important subsistence activities or valued plants and animals as seen through the eyes of the artisan. Caution must be exercised in interpreting artistic expressions, as these may incorporate attritubes associated with the plant or animal, or be stylistically modified so that exact identification is difficult and, when attempted, may be misleading.

In addition to spears, traps and snares are methods frequently used, particularly for catching small game. These are often made of perishable materials, such as plant fibers or sinew, and thus archeological examples are rarely preserved.

Stationary traps, on the other hand, may be quite noticeable in the landscape. These traps may act as a funnel to direct herd animals into a corral or fish into an enclosure. Traps or wiers of this sort are generally made by constructing stone walls or wood and brush barriers and often incorporate, or are aligned with, natural features. When these are used in animal drives, the funnel may direct the animals over a cliff, thereby killing them.

A herd animal drive and kill site may sometimes be possible to painstakingly reconstruct from an assemblage of animal remains. A good example of such detective work is that of the bison kill at the Olsen-Chubbuck site. Factors of the terrain, positions of the bison skeletons in respect to the terrain and to one another, and the completeness of the individual skeletons were all considered in reconstructing what Wheat (1972) described persuasively as a Paleo-Indian bison drive.

As can be seen from the previous discussion, there are only a few basic animal capture techniques. These have been modified in an almost infinite number of ways, thus adapting them to catch effectively each of the many animals that have been used in prehistoric times. The modifications that make the weapon successful are those that take into account the behavioral and physical characteristics of the prey species and capitalize on each animal's vulnerability.

AGRICULTURE

Of all the subsistence activities, agriculture and animal husbandry may leave the most permanent marks on the landscape. The management of water by the construction of drainage canals and ridged fields or irrigation systems can be seen many centuries after they were built. Terraced fields in regions with steep relief reduce problems of erosion and allow controlled irrigation and farming on a horizontal surface. Ridged fields that allow for drainage persist as a prominent feature of the present topography (Denevan 1970).

In the precipitous Andes terraces and irrigation systems that were constructed in prehistoric times are still in use. In this same area, corrals built throughout many centuries for the domesticated herds of llamas and alpacas are a prominent feature of the landscape. Prehistoric fish ponds can also be detected long after they were last used for raising selected fishes (Kikuchi 1976).

New techniques in aerial photography have greatly expanded our ability to see these ancient features in the modern landscape (Vogt 1974; Williams and Carter 1976). Infrared photography, stereoscopic pairs of photographs, computer programming of vegetation types, and other developments of the Earth Resources Technology Satellite have all advanced this technology. With these advances, remnants of large-scale alterations in the landscape related to human subsistence activities are revealed.

Artifacts most often directly associated with agricultural activities are

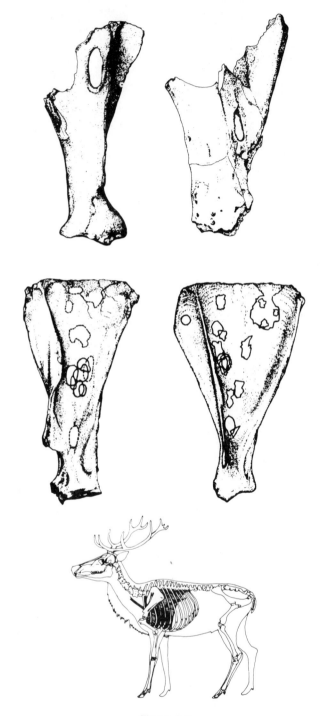

Figure 6-7

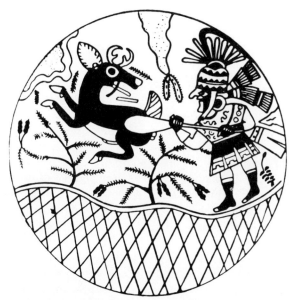

Figure 6-8. A fine line Mochica drawing of a deer hunt using a hunting net (reprinted from *Moche art and iconography* by permission of the author Christopher B. Donnan 1976:104).

stone, shell, or bone axes of various types used in land clearing. Microscopic analysis of the wear on stone or bone tools may reflect the texture of the material worked by the tool. If this material is coarse and gritty, as soil would be, it would leave broad scratches perpendicular to the working edge of the tool. On the other hand, if the material is soft and pliable, such as a hide, it will polish the working surface of the tool (Keeley and Newcomer 1977; Semenov 1957). Wooden tools used in planting, such as dibble sticks or wooden hafts for stone tools, are rarely preserved.

Further insight into prehistoric agricultural practices can be gained from such inscriptions as the hieroglyphics that survive in the Mexican Codices and stellae that express historical accounts and calendrical notations. The preoccupation with the calendar is interesting from the standpoint of scheduling subsistence activities as well as other events. The association of animals with the days of the month also reflects the significance of these animals and their attributes in the Aztec and Maya cosmic view. Another way the human memory was aided was by quipus, sets of knotted strings

◄━**Figure 6-7.** Repeated finds of injuries found in the scapula of red deer from the Mesolithic of Denmark. Two scapulae at top show healed fractures; two scapulae in middle show all of the examples of injuries superimposed on one scapula (dotted line: healed fractures; solid line: unhealed fractures); the outline drawing of the stag shows the position of the scapula in relation to the vital organs (reprinted by permission of North-Holland Press and the author from *Bone injuries caused by human weapons* by Nanna Noe-Nygaard 1975:157–158).

that quantify, among other things, herd and agricultural production. The significance of most quipus is still locked in the memories of the Incan messengers, who used these in helping to keep track of the economic affairs of the Inca Empire.

Other sources of information that provide insight into Indian life and foodways at the time of Spanish contact are commentaries written and illustrated at the period of adjustment between the two very different cultures. Famous among these are the letters of Cortes to Charles V, the accounts of Incan history by Garcilaso de la Vega, illustrations by Guaman Poma de Ayala, Fray Diego de Landa's descriptions of Maya life, the history of Mexico by Fray Bernadino de Sahagun, and Gonzalo Fernandez de Oviedo's account of the West Indies. Later accounts of travellers and explorers, such as Catlin, Bartram, Humboldt, Darwin, and Bates, provide insight into a way of life that has long since disappeared. Finally, documents from the Colonial period, such as lists of shipments of foods, trading post and farm inventories, and both official and private letters, can augment the data that is recovered archeologically. The types of descriptive and pictorial sources briefly listed here may not only support the interpretation based on the archeological data but may also supply information that would have no tangible evidence, thus allowing a fuller understanding of a past way of life.

FOOD PROCESSING

PLANT FOODS

Artifacts indirectly associated with agriculture or gathering are those that have been related to each of the many steps involved in preparing plant products for consumption. In the processing of corn (*Zea mays*), for example, a whole series of tools were used to prepare corn meal. Many of these tools and techniques may have accompanied the spread of this most important New World domestic plant. In husking dry corn, a pointed needle was widely used to split the shuck and remove the ear of corn. Farmers in Mexico from Sinaloa on the Pacific Coast, the Central highlands of Oaxaca, to Vera Cruz on the Gulf Coast still use a pointed tool called a *piscadore,* made from a sharpened deer metapodial, to split open the cornhusks (Figure 6.9). Similar tools with the same type of wear pattern are found as a universal household tool of the early Mesoamerican village (Flannery 1976). A tool that functions the same way but was made of bear bone was used by the Iroquois (Figure 6.9), and one made of a sharpened stick is used by the Vilcanota peasants of the Andes (Gade 1975; Waugh 1973). Similarly universal tools are a hand-held grinding stone and a stone mortar used together

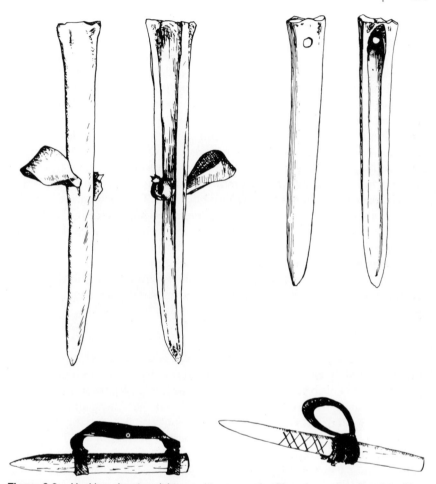

Figure 6-9. Husking pins: top right, a contemporary husking pin or piscadore from Vera Cruz, Mexico; top left, one from Sinaloa, Mexico (both are made from deer metapodia and drawn by Lynn C. Balck); bottom, Iroquois husking pins (by Lynn C. Balck from a photograph of a specimen in the National Museum of Canada in Ottawa.)

to grind the kernels of corn. The *mano* and *metate* are widespread Middle and South American tools with great antiquity and have usually been associated with the grinding of corn. A muller and mealing slab that function in the same way were used in prehistoric times by the Iroquois. A wooden mortar and pestle were widely used throughout North America. Equally widespread and with comparable antiquity are pots and jars used to store grain and other foods.

Another important crop widespread throughout the humid tropics of

America is manioc (*Manihot esculenta*). Associated with this root crop are also specific procedures for processing. The tubers are usually peeled, washed, and then grated, often on a board in which stone teeth are inserted. The resulting flour is cooked on a ceramic griddle. It is these durable small stone-flake teeth from the grating board and the pottery griddle that have been used to infer manioc cultivation, since the manioc itself is seldom preserved.

Caution must be used in interpreting any one of the implements just mentioned as evidence of corn or manioc cultivation. Each of these tools could equally well have been used for other purposes. Grinding is a necessary step in reducing many foods to a state in which they can be cooked or eaten (Carter 1977; DeBoer 1975; Kraybill 1977). Griddles, variously called *comales* when associated with corn and *budares* when associated with manioc, may have several functions. Therefore, the recovery of a whole complex of tools associated with the processing of a particular food strengthens the case that can be made for the prehistoric use of this food. Clearly biological remains of this food (see Chapter 7) or changes wrought by it in the human skeletons (see Chapter 6) will further support the interpretation.

DAMAGED BONE

Marks on bone are testimony of the wear and tear to which they have been subjected. Many of these marks are quite distinctive and indicate the types of treatment to which the bone was subjected. White, fresh breaks or scars are usually the result of accidental breakage during excavation or handling. A dendritic pattern on the bone or pitting and flaking of bone surface may be attributed to the chemical action of the soil and its destructive forces on bone. Grooves on the surface of bone that do not differ in color from the rest of the bone were made on the bone before it was deposited in the refuse. Such grooves may be the result of intentional modification of the bone preparatory to making a tool or ornament, or they may be the by-product of use of the bone or scars produced during the butchering or skinning process. Tool manufacture, particularly when it has progressed beyond the initial stage, can be recognized by the pattern of groove marks on the bone. A frequent early step in the procedure is repeated scoring of the bone, either lengthwise, preparatory to splitting the long bone, or circumferential scoring and ultimate breaking to separate the ends of the long bone from the shaft. As the production of the tool proceeds, the cut surface or the entire bone may be smoothed and polished. The care with which a bone tool is made is clearly different from the technique used in making a temporary tool (Sadek-Kooros 1972, 1975). Temporary tools are fractured in a way that results in a piece or pieces of bone that can be used without further modification. Repeated fragments of bone with the same shape and abrasion or wear marks are an indication of the production and use of temporary tools. Scars on bones resulting from butchering and skinning also tend to occur in a frequently repeated pattern (Guilday, Parmalee, and Tanner 1962). This pattern relates to anatomical features where the skin attaches closely to the skeleton, such as around the skull and feet, and must be cut to be removed and joints that are cut to disarticulation the carcass.

Grooves and scarring on bone can also be made by animals leaving equally distinctive alterations. Two animals that frequently are associated with human habitation and that gnaw on bones are dogs and rodents. Dogs typically gnaw the articulating end of bones leaving them ragged and pitted with small conical pits made by the dogs' pointed teeth (Figure 6.10). Usually, at least the dense shaft of larger long bones are not destroyed. It is of

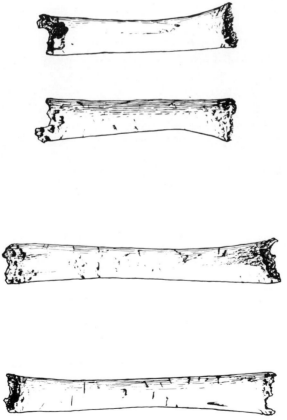

Figure 6-10. Marks left on bone chewed by a dog (drawn by Lynn C. Balck).

course a matter of speculation what bones may have been completely consumed or dragged away. Rodents gnaw bones with their two sets of opposing incisors. These incisors usually leave two rows of tiny parallel grooves very close together along the shaft of a bone (Figure 6.11). This results in a sharp ridge of bone between the rows of grooves where the upper and lower incisors met.

BROKEN BONE

Bones may become broken at any time between the capture of the animal and the study of their remains. Again, as with scars on bone, if the break is white and clean it is likely to be of recent origin. Otherwise, the bone may be broken in the process of preparing meat for food, particularly in the process of extracting marrow, purposely broken for a temporary tool, or broken subsequent to deposit through compaction or redeposition. Distinguishing between these is not easy. A regular pattern of breaks and evidence of use of bone fragments may be interpreted as the result of production of temporary tools. Certain skeletal elements would lend themselves more readily to the production of a tool. Breaks resulting from marrow extraction are only likely on long bones of large mammals. Likewise, removal of the brain requires breaking only the skull. Through the process of boiling or roasting, some of the organic material in bone is destroyed, making the bone more brittle and thereby less resistant to breakage.

Bones also differ in their innate resistance to abnormal stress. Small, compact, rounded bones, such as the tarsals and carpals of deer, are much more likely to withstand the wear and tear of time than slender fragile bones

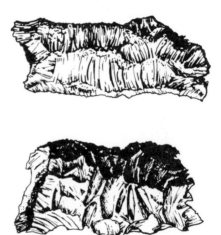

Figure 6-11. Marks left on bone chewed by a rodent (drawn by Lynn C. Balck).

in a bird skeleton. Thus, many factors can contribute to the breakage of organic material before recovery and study by archeologists.

BURNED BONE

Burning of bones may result from their use as a fuel, as a by product of roasting, or from disposal in a hearth. Burned bone ranges in color from white through grays and blues to black, depending on the completeness of its combustion. The destruction of the organic material in bone through burning makes the bone brittle and shrinks it from 5 to 15% in size and 50% in weight. Remnants of cremations are usually highly fragmented, often through purposeful destruction of the burned bone, and often much of the bone is white in color, suggesting complete oxidation. Charring of bone during roasting is confined to the exposed ends of the bone not protected from the fire by meat. The bone will appear partially blackened.

FAUNAL AND FLORAL ASSEMBLAGES

The presence of particular species of animal and plant remains may reveal much about the subsistence of which they are a remnant. The species composition of an archeologically associated faunal assemblage will indicate in broad terms some of the subsistence techniques that were used, for example, the relative importance of hunting as opposed to fishing. The habitat preference and seasonal availability of the species represented may also suggest what habitats were exploited and when during the year. The behavior of the species may provide clues to the means by which they can be obtained. The condition of these biological remains in themselves can show evidence of how the animal was caught or how the food was prepared and eaten. Butchering, roasting, and chewing may all leave their telltale marks. These and other significances of the species represented in archeological context will be discussed in detail in the following chapter.

Biological Material **7**
Used for Food

The habit of creating concentrated patches of food refuse and abandoned artifacts is amongst the basic features of behaviour that distinguishes the human animal from other primates. The habit has created a trail of litter that leads back through the Pleistocene and can provide an extremely important source of evidence regarding the evolution of human behaviour. Systematic archaeological study of the long term features of this garbage record is still in its infancy and yet it is already apparent that it is far from being a trivial pursuit. [Isaac 1971:278]

VERTEBRATE REMAINS

Foods are organic material composed of edible plant and animal tissue. This is true, notwithstanding synthetic foods and food supplements that have come into vogue particularly in the twentieth century. The inedible or undigested residue of prehistoric food provide some of the best clues to past foodways. Different foods leave different remains. What is left depends in part on the durability of the inedible or undigestible parts. As described earlier (Chapter 1), many factors, both human and environmental, will affect both the preservation and the recovery of these organic materials.

Once recovered, these remains must be identified and studied so that their role as a remnant of a former food may be understood. The basic procedure of identification is the same for all organic material. Ultimately, the reconstruction of the prehistoric foodway will be based on the identification of all faunal and floral material recovered and will draw upon an understanding of the ecology of the plants and animals used, as well as that of the user.

Bibliographies to research in zooarcheology include references to far more studies than can be discussed here. The annotated bibliography by Angress and Reed (1962) is a guide to further reading on topics of animal domestication. A bibliography of zooarcheology in eastern North America (Bogan and Robison 1978) lists references pertaining to studies of animal remains excavated from archeological sites.

IDENTIFICATION

We understand the living world in the light of identified and described organisms and processes. Taxonomic descriptions, revisions, and keys are the standard sources for identification of biological material. These sources include the original descriptions, subsequent revisions, and regional and local faunal reports. A broad regional coverage of major taxonomic groups is provided by the relatively inexpensive Peterson Field Guide Series to the different plant and animal groups. Other sources exist that provide information about Latin American flora and fauna, such as Meyer de Schauensee's book about South American birds (1970), Cabrera and Yepe's book on the mammals (1960), and Randall's guide to Caribbean reef fishes (1968). More local reports of the taxonomy and distribution of a vertebrate class or family must be relied upon as guides to the faunal assemblage that may be expected to occur in a given area. Such published sources give the scientific names of groups of organisms and the characteristics by which they may be distinguished. These distinguishing characteristics or key characters are usually external features of the whole plant or animal and certain internal structures, such as those related to feeding or reproduction.

When internal parts of an organism, such as the skull and postcranial skeleton, are to be identified, published keys and descriptions are less readily available. Thus, fragmentary remains of animals associated with archeological materials are identified by comparison with previously identified specimens. This is best done by a process of elimination starting with the broadest taxonomic classification, such as phylum and class, and working down to genus and species. The characteristics of the skeleton and teeth of the broad taxonomic groups are described in general texts, such as *Vertebrate Paleontology* by Romer (1945). Reference must be made to increasingly specialized texts to aid in the identification of the lower taxons. Positive identification to the generic or specific level must be made by comparison of the unidentified material with a series of identified specimens. These comparative specimens would, of course, have been identified with reference to the more standard taxonomic keys prior to their preparation as comparative skeletons.

An example may help to illustrate this procedure. A vertebrate faunal sample excavated from the coastal plain of the southeastern United States includes bones of what is judged to be a medium-sized mammal. Associated with these bones are teeth that are high-crowned, typical of a herbivore. The types of animals that would fulfill these qualifications would be rabbits, muskrat, porcupine, marmot, and nutria. The natural range in distribution of porcupines is too far north at the present time, although they existed in the Southeast during the Pleistocene. The nutria has been very recently introduced, and prehistoric occurrence in the Southeast is improbable. The present range of these animals should by no means exclude them entirely from consideration, as animal distributions change through time; however, the more likely candidates are rabbit, marmot, and beaver (Hall and Kelson 1959; Lowery 1974; Miller and Kellogg 1955). Next, one can compare the bones to the illustrations in the guide to North American mammal skeletons by Gilbert (1973). This may suggest that the bones in question are similar to those of a rabbit. Verification of such a tentative identification must be made by comparison with a series of prepared comparative skeletons, which are available in many museum research collections. Use of museum collections must be negotiated with the curators of those collections.

The manual of mammalian osteology by Gilbert (1973), which has been mentioned, and other similar manuals, such as those by Olsen (1964) and the atlas of European mammal bones by Schmid (1972), are exceedingly helpful for the initial tentative identification of skeletal material of North American mammals. An illustrated guide with keys to aid in the identification of bird bones from North American archeological sites is presently being prepared (Gilbert, Martin, and Savage n.d.). Comparable guides for the identification of skeletal material for other vertebrate groups and for mammals of South America are not presently available. A number of excellent, well-illustrated osteological studies of small, taxonomic groups, such as the Mexican Macaws (Hargrave 1970), the chicken and American grouse (Hargrave 1972), the domestic turkey (Harvey, Kaiser, and Rosenberg 1968), Florida snakes (Auffenberg 1963), and domestic dog (Miller 1964), are nonetheless very useful sources. Of larger taxonomic scope and often helpful in narrowing down identification to the familial level is Gregory's (1933/1959) book on fish skulls. At the present time, published guides in comparative osteology illustrated in sufficient detail and of broad enough geographic and taxonomic scope do not fulfill all the needs encountered in the identification of vertebrate remains. This leaves reference to a comparative collection as the most viable procedure for fragmentary skeletal identification. It may be desirable to establish a comparative collection specifically for one's research needs and for continued access. Such an endeavor should not be entered into lightly. Preparation of a comparative collection is a time consuming and costly enterprise. A variety of techniques that may be used to prepare comparative skeletons are described by Gilbert (1973). More importantly, complex federal, state, and foreign regulations govern the collection and possession of animals and their parts (see the Appendix). These laws restrict what animals may be taken, when during the year, and how they are collected. An easy way of collecting animals is to pick up highway fatalities. However, caution must be exercised here, too, as it is illegal to possess an endangered species or migratory bird, even if they are found dead. The legal complexities of collecting in a foreign country and importing the collected materials are greatly increased. The details of these laws depend on the countries involved. Before embarking on a skeleton-collection project, it is recommended that the legal aspects be thoroughly reviewed.

In the identification of fragmentary faunal remains, the details of the characteristics of teeth and skeletal elements that are used differ for each element and each vertebrate class; however, the general types of characteristics that may be relied on are similar. These diagnostic characteristics are the shape and size of a skeletal element; the shape of the articulating surface; the position, size, and shape of foramena and muscle scars; and the pattern of cusps and roots and the height of the crown in teeth. In the identification of a skeletal element, a combination of a number of key or diagnostic characteristics are used to set the element of one species apart from all others.

The degree to which the unidentified element must correspond with the comparable element of a comparative specimen depends on a number of factors. One of these factors is the innate variability of individuals within a population that is particularly evident in some taxonomic groups. Populations of a species may also differ, one from another. Differences related to age and sex are perhaps most clearly reflected in the skeleton and dentition. Equally profound are the differences in size and proportions of animals that have been subject to human manipulation in the process of domestication. Examples of the changes wrought by domestication have been clearly analyzed for several Eurasian domesticates (Higham 1968). Finally, characteristic changes in bone and teeth result from a variety of congenital malformations, injuries, and diseases. Because of these many sources of variation, comparison of unidentified specimens with a series of comparative specimens is essential.

INDIVIDUAL AND POPULATION VARIATION

Variation between populations of a species and individuals within a population are often reflected in skeletal material as differences in size. Well-known size trends, such as increase in size, correlated with increasingly high latitudes exist in warm-blooded vertebrates (Ricklefs 1973:134). Those characteristics related to size and proportion, such as an absolute increase in measurements, have a concomitant increase in muscle-scar development with robustness.

AGE CHANGES

The changes in the skeleton related to age are not only an increase in size, although this of course is basic, but there are also changes in the texture of the bone tissue during this process of growth. Bone of young reptiles, birds, and mammals has a fibrous texture, and suture joints as in the skull, turtle shell, and between the diaphysis and epiphysis are unfused. The fusion of the epiphysis to the diaphysis in mammals follows a regular sequence related to the growth pattern of each mammalian species. The actual age of fusion, however, varies with the physical condition and sex of the animal (Gilbert 1973:49). In some groups in which growth continues throughout much of the animal's life, fusion may only be complete in relatively old age. Bone becomes longer, thicker, and denser by appositional growth and will change in proportion by absorption and remodeling (Weinmann and Sicher 1947). Muscle scars on bone, the development of bone crests for attachment of heavy muscle masses, mark bones of mature animals. Increased rugosity of the surface of some bone, for example some turtle shells (*Chrysemys scripta, Trionyx ferox, Chelydra serpentina*) and alligator (*Alligator mississipiensis*), skulls, and scutes, is also correlated with increased size and age. In some fishes pneumatic bones, sometimes called Tilly bones, form with advancing age. Pneumatic bone typically forms on the neural spines and neural crest and less frequently on the pterygeophores and cleithrum. It appears externally as an amorphous rounded swelling in the bone and internally it is vasicular like hardened froth.

The eruption, replacement, and wear of teeth in mammals may also be correlated with age. As with epiphysial fusion, the precise ages of the stages in this sequence differ for each species. The milk dentition erupts in orderly fashion and foreshadows the form of the permanent dentition. As the milk dentition becomes worn, it will in a predictable sequence be replaced by the permanent dentition. At the same time, there might be worn milk teeth and new unworn permanent teeth in the mouth, which may cause confusion in determining the age of the animal. Once the permanent dentition is in place it, too, will become worn.

This progression of tooth eruption and wear follows a precise enough pattern that these stages may indicate the age of the animal within a range of variation. This range increases with the increased age of the animal. As an animal gets older, the permanent dentition is subjected to foods that differ greatly in the amount that they will abrade the teeth. Stone-ground corn meal, in which is incorporated fine stone particles, is well known to abrade human teeth quickly. Such meal is by no means the only abrasive food. As an animal gets older, the wear on its teeth by abrasive foods will be accumulated, and its age will be increasingly difficult to estimate. Stages in eruption and average wear have been outlined for deer (Severinghaus 1949) as well as other animals of economic interest.

Incremental structures preserved in the hard tissues of vertebrates can also indicate the animal's age. Such incremental structures are layers of dentine in mammalian teeth, growth rings in fish otoliths, opercula, scales, fin rays, and vertebrae (Casteel, 1976a,b; Chaplin 1971). Most of these growth rings result from alternating rapid and slow growth, reflecting annual environmental pulses. In some geographic regions, these seasonal pulses may be less marked or have less effect on these incremental structures, making them difficult to use in assessing age. In every case, correlations between chronological age and incremental structures must be established for each species by examination of a series of individual specimens of known age.

SEXUAL DIFFERENCES

Sexually determined characteristics also are manifest in the skeleton. Male members of the higher vertebrates, mammals and birds, often attain a greater size, which of course may be seen in the larger, more robust skeletons of fully mature individuals. In addition to the differences in size range between males and females, a number of structures related to secondary sexual characteristics may be observed in skeletons. Most prominent of these is antler development in deer. Antlers develop and are annually shed in male deer. Reindeer are an exception in that antlers develop in both sexes. Each successive year, the newly grown antlers of a given buck may be larger, although this development is modified by many factors. The size of the tusks or canines of pigs and a number of other mammals differ between the sexes. The males of many species of carnivores and rodents have bracula or penis bones. Another familiar sex-related structure is the spur which develops on the tarsometatarsus or lower leg of gallinaceous cocks, such as chickens and turkeys (Hargrave 1972:20–22). Terrestrial turtles (*Terrapene carolina* and *Gopherus polyphemus*) have modifications which in part answer the question posed by Ogden Nash (1941):[1] "The turtle lives 'twixt plated decks which practically conceal its sex. I think it clever of the turtle in such a fix to be so fertile." To facilitate breeding the posterior half of the plastron of male box turtles and tortoises is concave to accommodate the curve of the female carapace. In addition, the anterior margin of the plastron of gopher tortoises projects and is used as a ram during courtship combat.

[1]Reprinted with the permission of Little, Brown and Company.

A type of bone related to sexual differences in the skeleton is known as medullary bone. This is loose disorganized deposits of bone on the interior of many of the long-bone shafts of most birds (Rick 1975). These deposits are laid down during the period of egg laying and are drawn upon for the production of egg shell. Medullary bone is, therefore, found primarily in females and confined to the egg-laying part of the reproductive cycle. The presence of medullary bone, therefore, can provide sexual and seasonal information (Figure 7.1).

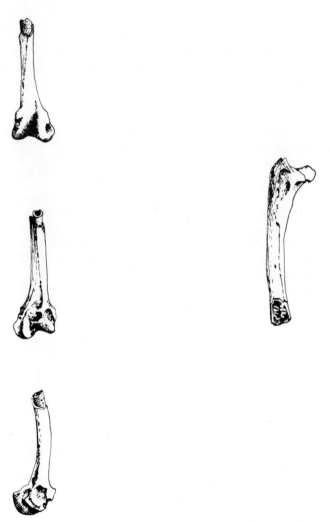

Figure 7-1. Example of the core of soft medullary bone within the shaft of a chicken femur. (drawn by Lynn C. Balck).

The degree to which any of these characteristics are expressed varies with the individual animal. Individual variation in the expression of qualitative and quantitative characteristics may be seen in all vertebrates; however, the range in these variations differs from one vertebrate group to another. Among the most highly variable animals are those that have been domesticated. Even prior to modern stock breeding, domesticates ranged widely in size, proportion, and characteristics, such as color and texture of the hair. This greater variability is seen as a result of human manipulation and selection of particular phenotypic characteristics in animals they have used. It is possible to maintain the observed ranges in domesticates while under human protection and in part relieved from the rigors of natural selection. Under the care and protection afforded a domestic animal, it may survive disease and injury affecting the hard tissues more readily than an animal in the wild. However, recent studies show that some wild animal populations may also sustain considerable trauma and survive (Maples, personal communication). Disease lesions and injuries usually appear as disorganized pitting or hypertrophy of the bone. The bone itself may often appear fibrous and as such distinguishable from normal adult tissue.

QUANTIFICATION

Animal remains are the data base of faunal analysis. Primary data derived from these remains are the raw counts, weights, and measurements of shell, bone, and tooth fragments recovered (Clason 1972). Primary data or basic data are direct quantification of identified material. These differ from secondary data, such as minimum numbers of individuals (see p. 123), and usable meat weight (see p. 126), which involve interpretation, extrapolation, or estimations based on the primary data.

SAMPLE SIZE

As with any scientific endeavor, sample size may alter the results. Often in archeological research, it is not possible to obtain as much material as is deemed desirable. The sample size will determine to some extent the type of interpretation of the data that will be feasible. How to determine what size sample is adequate is also not simple. A number of different criteria could be used, depending on the focus of the research. If the concern of the research is to reconstruct butchering techniques, an adequate sample would have to include the full range of butchering scars. Another guide that could be used to measure the adequacy of a sample is the number of species represented.

The line of reasoning that may be followed in establishing a guide for measuring the adequacy of a sample is: (a) determine the point of diminishing returns at which few new species are added to the faunal assemblage with the identification of additional minimum numbers of individuals; (b) correlate the minimum numbers of individuals with the number of identifiable specimens; and (c) calculate the portion of the faunal sample that is identifiable. An example may help to illustrate this procedure.

In a comparison between minimum numbers of individuals, computed for each cultural unit using Chaplin's formula (1971:16), and number of species represented in 73 faunal samples, one sees a sharp increase in the number of species until the sample is composed of about 200 minimum numbers of individuals, after which few new species are added (Figure 7.2). In other words, a sample of 200 minimum number of individuals would be large enough to include most of the species used at that site, and, therefore, by adding to the sample relatively few new species will be identified. This correlation is based on faunal samples from sites located on the circum-Caribbean coastal plain. The people occupying these sites had access to animal resources from a variety of aquatic and terrestrial habitats, which resulted in a high species diversity. For those sites with faunal assemblages that have a low species diversity, such as most sites located in northern latitudes or at high altitudes or those with specialized diets, this criterion of adequacy would not be valid.

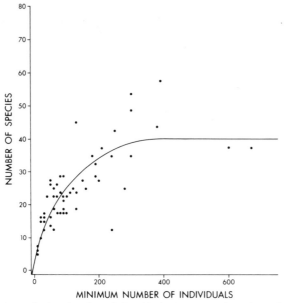

Figure 7-2. A graph showing the relationship between number of species and minimum number of individuals in circum-Caribbean faunal samples.

The relationship between minimum numbers of individuals and number of identifiable specimens is a direct one, except when samples are very small (Casteel 1976–1977). The comparison between number of identifiable specimens and minimum number of individuals suggests that a sample of approximately 1400 identifiable specimens are needed to generate at least 200 individuals in this sample of sites (Figure 7.3). A similar study by Casteel (1976–1977) indicates that, in a correlation between minimum numbers of individuals and identifiable specimens, there are as many as 44 identified specimens for each individual. He further demonstrates that small samples are subject to more biases in the index of minimum number of individuals than are large samples. A great deal of variation between sites may be expected. The figures given here may serve as a rough guide, particularly in choosing an adequate sample from a very large collection or assessing the reliability of a small sample.

The third variable in determining the adequacy of a sample is the portion of the sample that is unidentifiable. The average portion that was found to be unidentifiable in these samples from Caribbean sites was 23% with a range from 3 to 51%.

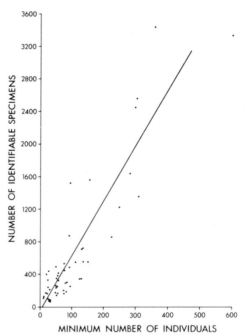

Figure 7-3. A graph comparing the minimum number of individuals and number of identifiable specimens from circum-Caribbean sites.

As indicated earlier, this procedure is included simply to serve as a guide to choosing an adequate sample from a very large collection or in assessing the reliability of a small sample. As reason would dictate, the larger the sample, the more accurately it should reflect the fauna of the site. Faunal analysis is, however, time consuming and this cost may sometimes have to be weighed in choosing the size sample to be studied.

PRIMARY DATA

A number of factors can bias the results of the primary data. These biases affecting the representation of the animal species used interfere with the accuracy with which the quantification reflects former patterns of animal use. As discussed earlier, recovery of faunal remains is rarely 100% successful. Whatever the thoroughness of the recovery might have been, the bone count as a measure of the numbers of different animals used can still be modified by several factors. Chief among these are the differences in the numbers of identifiable skeletal elements in different species. Not only do the species belonging to different classes vary a great deal in this respect, but so do the species within one class. Common representatives of the three major vertebrate classes, the dog (*Canis familiaris*), turkey (*Meleagris gallopavo*), and snook (*Centropomis undecimalis*), have approximately the same number of easily identifiable skeletal elements ranging from 29 to 47. Whereas other mammals and fish, for example, the armadillo (*Dasypus novemcinctus*) and gar (*Lepisosteus osseus*), have in the neighborhood of 2000 identifiable elements when scales and bony scutes are considered. Differences in species representation based on the count of fragments also result from breakage of bones. The amount of breakage varies from site to site and within parts of a single site and also differs between the skeletons of different species because of innate differences in their fragility or the use to which they were put. These variables which can affect the counts of identified and unidentified bone fragments must be kept in mind when evaluating these primary data.

Fragment Count

The primary data should include all the pertinent direct observations that may be made. Initially, identification is made of each fragment to the lowest taxon that can be demonstrated morphologically. In most cases, this leaves portions of each faunal assemblage identified only as mammal, bird, reptile, or fish, and a portion that can only be identified as vertebrate bone. The identified skeletal elements or portions of elements are recorded, indicating the name of the element, portion present (distal, proximal, and/or shaft), and the side (right or left). Characteristics of age, sex, and modifications, such as burning, gnawing, butchering marks, and polishing from use or steps in tool or ornament manufacture, are also recorded.

Bone Measurement

Another type of basic or primary data is measurements of the bone and tooth remains. Measurements are taken for several reasons which will be discussed in greater detail later. Measurements may be used to help in distinguishing between different species, between domestic and wild forms (Clason 1972; Higham 1968), between breeds of a domestic form (Haag 1948), and between sexes (Chaplin 1971). Measurements may also be used as a guide to estimates of the animal's height or weight (Clason 1972; Casteel 1974). These measurements are taken with vernier or dial calipers in metric units. Uniformity in taking these measurements is important so that the measurements may be compared with those taken on other remains. A guide to measurements of skeletal elements of mammals and birds is presented by von den Driesch (1976). Although this is an exhaustive guide, occasions may occur when other measurements must be taken to gain specific information. Whatever measurements are taken, a balance must be achieved between the most useful measurement to take, in terms of variability or correlation with increased size of the whole animal, and a measurement that is practical, one that is taken on a skeletal part that is usually, or at least often, preserved.

Bone Weight

Weight of the faunal remains is the final type of data that are considered basic. As with the other types of primary data, the accuracy of bone weight as a reflection of the weights of the bones of animals used in the past can be modified in a number of ways. The adherence of dirt or the mineralization of the bone would increase its weight. On the other hand cooking or burning decreases the weight of bone by as much as 50% (von den Driesch 1976).

Despite these difficulties, weights of skeletal material can provide insight into animal use not easily gained by other methods. The basis of this insight is the biological relationship between the weight of supporting tissue and body weight. This relationship is allometric and can be described by an allometric equation for the slope and intercept of the least squares logarithmic regression line (Prange, Anderson, and Rahn 1979). The mechanical parameters suggested by this allometry is that the skeletons of large animals are proportionately more massive than those of small animals, and that the skeleton mass of birds is not reduced as an adaptation for flight, although the weight is internally redistributed (Prange et al. 1979). The practical application of these equations is obvious, as one can use them to predict body weight if the skeletal weight of an animal is known. However, if one has the weight of only part of the skeleton of an animal, this part will scale as though it was a smaller animal. Nevertheless, weights of skeletal remains have a closer relationship to body weights of the animals used and by extrapolation to usable meat weight than do the other basic data, fragment counts. A sample of bones from the La Chimba site in the northern highlands of Ecuador, which was composed primarily of rabbit and deer, may be used to illustrate this. As can be seen in Table 7.1, the relative magnitudes between these data are reversed—rabbit is represented by three times as many identifiable fragments as deer, but these fragments contribute only 12% of the weight of these remains.

The question then is, what do these data signify? Do either the fragment count or the weight of remains relate to the number of animals used, or the amount of meat these animals provided? As indicated earlier, these data may be subject to inaccuracy in reflecting the animals that were used. A number of different methods that attempt to more accurately approximate the relative use of the identified animals have been advocated. These methods are all estimations and as such must be treated as secondary data.

SECONDARY DATA

Estimates of Minimum Numbers of Individuals

The most well known and widely used secondary data are the estimated minimum number of individuals represented in a sample (Clason 1972). This basic concept was introduced to most American archeologists in White's (1953a,b) pioneering papers in zooarcheology. Estimates of minimum numbers of individuals are computed by counting the most abundant elements. For example, if a sample includes three right and two left dentaries of a species, it is estimated that at least three individuals of that species are represented. However, if one of the left dentaries came from a very young animal, younger than all of the other individuals, one might conclude that four individuals were represented.

Since the publication of White's papers, many refinements on this basic method have been advocated (Casteel 1977; Chaplin 1971; Grayson 1973). The two variables affecting the estimations of the minimum number of individuals represented in archeological material are the following: (a) the excavation units that are used in determining numbers of individuals; and (b) the number of factors, such as age, size, and sex, that are taken into account to amplify the count of the most numerous element. The excavation units frequently used to form the basis of analysis are: (a) the arbitrary excavation unit (maximum distinction method of Grayson [1973]); (b) the cultural unit or natural stratum of a multicomponent site; or (c) the entire sample from the site as a whole (minimum distinction method of Grayson [1973]). Circumstances of excavation may dictate which method is prefer-

TABLE 7.1.
Primary and Secondary Data from Faunal Samples from the La Chimba Site, Ecuador.

| | Primary data | | | | Secondary data | | | |
Species	Number of bone and tooth fragments	%	Weight of fragments (kg)	%	Minimum numbers of individuals	%	Biomass[a] (kg)	%
Rabbit (*Sylvilagus brasiliensis*)	6658	69.2	4.1201	11.6	424	70.8	47.698	13.5
Deer (*Odocoileus virginianus*) and other cervids	2968	30.8	31.2979	88.4	176	29.4	306.479	86.5
Total	9626		35.418		599		354.177	

[a]Skeletal weight (kg) = .061 (body weight [kg])$^{1.09}$ (Prange *et al.* 1979).

able. A feature, such as a burial or storage pit, would be important to analyze as a discrete part of the excavated material. Caution, however, must be used in using arbitrary excavation levels as the unit for calculating an estimate of minimum numbers of individuals, because the bones of a single individual could easily be spread over several proveniences. At the other extreme, in that the resulting values are the most conservative, are calculations of estimated minimum numbers of individuals based on the entire faunal assemblage from a site. In a single component site, this would be the most valid unit of analysis to avoid the danger of recounting an animal whose skeleton is distributed over several arbitrary excavation units. However, in analysis based on the entire faunal sample of a multicomponent site, this method would mask any changes in animal use during cultural occupations. Calculation of estimates of minimum numbers of individuals based on the fauna of each cultural component may reveal changes in animal use and at the same time avoid overrepresenting an animal whose skeleton is dispersed in more than one arbitrary level.

A great range in results is achieved by different methods in calculating minimum numbers of individuals from a given faunal sample. The most conservative estimates result from simply counting the rights and lefts of the most commonly represented skeletal element and using the highest value as the estimated minimum number of individuals. This estimate, however, may be amplified by pairing the right and left elements according to characteristics such as size, age, and sex. This method is expressed in Chaplin's (1971:74) formula, which is as follows:

$$GMT = C^t/2 + D^t$$

where

GMT = grand minimum number of animals;
C^t = the total number of comparable paired elements;
D^t = the total number of dissimilar elements.

Greatly expanded values can result from using the formula proposed by Krantz (1968:286), which is as follows:

$$N = \frac{R^2 + L^2}{2P}$$

where

N = number of animals in the original population;
R = total number of right elements found;
L = total number of left elements found;
P = number of pairs of elements established.

This method attempts to estimate the number of animals in the original population. (A comparison of these two methods can be found in Casteel [1977].)

Yet another method proposed by Perkins (1973:267–369) is the relative abundance of species in a faunal assemblage based on the ratio of the number of specimens of each species unaffected by cultural and preservational factors identified in an assemblage by the potential number of diagnostic elements of each species. The difficulty with this method is in determining which elements would not be affected by either cultural or preservational factors.

The two methods for estimating minimum numbers of individuals most frequently used are (a) the count of the most numerous skeletal element; and (b) this count amplified by matching pairs of elements according to characteristics of size, age, and sex. These estimates are not viewed as absolute numbers, except in the rare case of excavation of an entire site, but form the basis for calculations of relative abundance of the represented species. The nature of archeological material is such that this relative abundance must be considered the relative abundance throughout the occupation sampled rather than a reflection of daily consumption or an average meal.

Biomass and Usable Meat Weights

One of the main objectives of the study of animal remains from archeological sites is to gain some insight into the types of animals used for prehistoric subsistence. Not only is it important to know what animals were used, but also how much food each could provide. A number of different methods have been proposed to estimate body weight from skeletal weight. This may be symptomatic of the difficulties in making these estimates and the relative inaccuracy of some of these methods. Five of these methods are described below.

White Method   Perhaps the oldest and most frequently used method is that described by White in a 1953 paper in which he listed mammals and birds that were commonly used, the average weight for each, and the percentage of the usable live weight. When these averages are applied to individuals from populations of smaller sized animals or young individuals, large errors result.

Smith (1975) proposed a refinement of this method for estimating live weight for white-tailed deer. The differences in size attributable to the sex and age of the animal are taken into consideration by Smith's method. The difficulties inherent in this method are that it is not always possible to assign age and sex to the individuals represented in a faunal sample, and that comparative data on size changes correlated with age and sex are, at this time, available only for deer.

Scaling—Dimensional Allometry   Another method is based on the innate relationships between linear dimensions and live body weight. Casteel (1974) has described a method of correlating a linear dimension of the skeleton with the animal's total live weight by using a least squares regression analysis. The equation: body weight $= b$ (chosen linear dimension)^a (where a is the slope and b the y-intercept of a log–log plot) is used. Casteel has used this method as a means of estimating the live weight of Sacramento Blackfish (*Orthodon microlepidotus*) and suckers (family Catostomidae) by measuring the centrum width of the posterior face of the precaudal vertebrae and the length of the otolith respectively (Table 7.2). Of somewhat broader application, but accompanied by less reliability, is a formula that shows the relationship between the anterior width of the atlas of teleost fishes and their body weight (Table 7.2). As further examples of this method, two other relationships between linear dimensions and body weight in mammals may be presented. Based on the rationale that supporting structures must be proportional to the weight they support in order to function, the greatest width of the femur head and the greatest breadth of the occipital condyles in mammals were correlated with body weight (Table 7.2). This method allows for quite accurate body-weight predictions, but two drawbacks are evident. First, to establish good correlations between linear dimensions and body weight, a large series of specimens with accurate body weight data must be available. Second, the linear measurement should be on a bone or tooth that is frequently found in measurable condition in faunal material (Figure 7.4).

Scaling—Skeletal Mass Allometry   A slightly different approach for estimating body weight from fragmentary skeletal remains is by a correlation of skeletal weight with body weight. This is based on the fundamental relationship that exists between the weight of supporting tissue and the total body weight. A number of studies of scaling have correlated body weight with the skeletal weight of a number of taxonomic groups (Pedley 1977; Prange *et al.* 1979; Reitz 1979; Reynolds and Karlotski 1977). (See Table 7.2 and Figure 7.5.)

As with other methods, however, problems in applying this method exist. One of the problems innate in the relationship between skeletal weight and body weight is that the two are not directly proportional. In other words, an animal half the body weight of another does not have a skeletal weight that is half the skeletal weight of the larger. Therefore, if one has half the skele-

TABLE 7.2.
Selected Allometric Formulas

1. Blackfish vertebrate to live weight
   $\log y = 2.4497 (\log x) + 0.9138; r = 0.987; N = 768$
   - $x =$ centrum width (mm) of precaudal vertebra of Sacramento blackfish (*Orthodon microlepidotus*)
   - $y =$ body weight (gm) (Casteel 1974)
2. Sucker otolith to live weight
   $\log y = 3.4288 (\log x) + 0.8845; r = 0.977; N = 89$
   - $x =$ otolith length (mm) of suckers (Castostomidae)
   - $y =$ body weight (gm) (Casteel 1974)
3. Teleost vertebrae to live weight
   $\log y = 2.047 (\log x) + 1.162; r = 0.85; r^2 = 0.72; N = 50$
   - $x =$ anterior width (mm) of the centrum of the atlas of bony fish
   - $y =$ body weight (gm)
4. Breadth of occipital condyles of terrestrial mammals to live weight
   $\log y = 3.2659 (\log x) - 0.9421; r = 0.98; r^2 = 0.96; N = 17$
   - $x =$ greatest breadth (mm) of occipital condyles in terrestrial mammals
   - $y =$ body weight (gm)
5. Width of femur head in terrestrial mammal to live weight
   $\log y = 2.5569 (\log x) + 0.8671; r = 0.98; r^2 = 0.96; N = 40$
   - $x =$ greatest diameter (mm) of the femur head in terrestrial mammals
   - $y =$ body weight (gm)
6. Mammal skeletal weight to live weight
   $\log y = 1.09 (\log x) - 1.2147; r = 0.99; N = 49$
   - $x =$ body weight (kg)
   - $y =$ skeletal weight (kg) (Prange *et al.* 1979)
7. Bird skeletal to live weight
   $\log y = 1.071 (\log x) - 1.1871; r = 0.99; N = 311$
   - $x =$ body weight (kg)
   - $y =$ skeletal weight (kg) (Prange *et al.* 1979)
8. Turtle skeletal weight to live weight
   $\log y = 0.5004 (\log x) + 0.4684; r = 0.68; r^2 = 0.46; N = 28$
   - $x =$ skeletal weight (kg)
   - $y =$ body weight (kg)
9. Snake skeletal weight to live weight
   $\log y = 1.0107 (\log x) + 1.1660; r = 0.98; r^2 = 0.96; N = 26$
   - $x =$ skeletal weight (kg)
   - $y =$ body weight (kg)
10. Elasmobranch skeletal (vertebrae and teeth) to live weight
    $\log y = 0.8613 (\log x) + 1.6846; r = 0.92; r^2 = 0.85; N = 17$
    - $x =$ skeletal weight (kg)
    - $y =$ body weight (kg)
11. Teleost skeletal weight to live weight
    $\log y = 0.8682 (\log x) + 1.1136; r = 0.87; r^2 = 0.76; N = 177$
    - $x =$ skeletal weight (kg)
    - $y =$ body weight (kg)

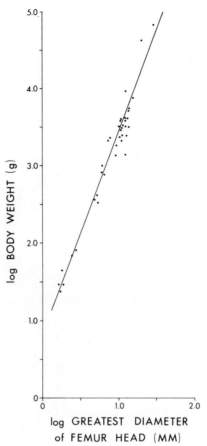

Figure 7-4. Relationship between the greatest diameter of the femur head (x) and body weight (y) of terrestrial mammals.

ton of an animal, the resulting body-weight estimate will not be exactly half the total body weight. Further inaccuracy will be introduced if the bone weight is very dirty, is mineralized, or the bone minerals are leached. Such changes affecting bone weight will, of course, be a factor influencing the accuracy of any method for which the basis of body-weight estimates is skeletal weight.

Percentage Method A method proposed by Reed (1963) is based on the assumption that the skeletal weight of mammals is 7.5% of body weight. This is, of course, an approximation, and other percentages, ranging from 5.6 to 9%, have been used. These estimates are the easiest to arrive at, but

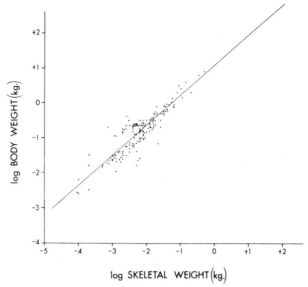

Figure 7-5. Relationship between the skeletal weight (x) and body weight (y) of teleost fishes.

this simplicity must be balanced by the relative inaccuracy of the results, which is inevitable when the allometric nature of this relationship is understood.

Proportional Method The last method is simply to set up a proportion of the skeletal weight with a known skeletal-weight–body-weight ratio for an animal of the same species (Ziegler 1973).

The accuracy with which these five methods estimate biomass can be assessed by testing these methods with comparative specimens of known weight. The average and the range in percentage of error in estimating the weight of 10 specimens is summarized in Table 7.3.

As may be seen, estimates of body weight using the White method may be very inaccurate. The greatest amount of deviation in actual weight comes from using an average weight for a species that is, of course, composed of young, small individuals and adults that vary in age and, therefore, size. This error is compounded when the average weights of reptiles and fishes are used, as these vertebrates continue to grow throughout adult life.

Much greater accuracy is achieved from the methods of scaling, by using correlations either between a dimension or between skeletal weight and body weight. As might be anticipated, the dimensional relationship of the breadth of the occipital condyles is more accurate in predicting body weight than is the width of the femur head, which is subject to variation related to different modes of locomotion.

The percentage and proportional methods are, on the average, less accurate methods of predicting body weight than the scaling methods.

In a similar comparison, Casteel (1978) tested the reliability of estimates of pig-meat weight determined from bone weights by variations of the scaling, percentage, and proportional methods. He reports even higher errors in the estimations derived by the percentage and proportional methods than are reported here. The error in estimation from using scaling formulas established for pig meat and pig soft-tissue weights correlated with bone weights are, however, even more accurate, ranging from .009 to 7%, than the test of the scaling-method formula for all terrestrial mammals presented here. A partial explanation for the high percentage of error observed by Casteel is that he introduced additional sources of error by estimating body weight and by estimating the amount of the body weight that was meat weight, thereby compounding the sources of an error.

An estimation is by definition an approximation, in this case the weight of biomass, and it has inherent error. The range in error of some of these techniques may be used as a guide (Table 7.3). If a further estimation is made to assess the amount of usable meat an animal could provide, the error is compounded. Such error is inevitable and must be recognized when attempts are made to calculate the potential yield of meat to the prehistoric diet based on fragmentary faunal remains.

TABLE 7.3.
The Average Error in Estimates of Body Weight Predicted by Different Methods

---

1. *White method:*
   Average weight of species under consideration
   $N = 10$, average 142.7%, range 1.9% to 839.6%
2. *Scaling—Dimensional allometry:*
   A. Width of femur head to live weight
      $N = 16$, average 26.6%, range 3.4% to 64.3%
   B. Breadth of occipital condyles in mammals to live weight
      $N = 16$, average 18.9%, range 3.1% to 52.8%
   C. Anterior width of atlas of any teleost to live weight
      $N = 10$, average 22.2%, range 0% to 47.1%
3. *Scaling—Skeletal mass allometry:*
   Terrestrial mammal skeletal weight to live weight
   $N = 10$, average 12.4%, range 1.4% to 25.8%
4. *Percentage method:*
   Assuming bone in mammals equals 7.5% of body weight
   $N = 10$, average 30.7%, range 1.9% to 66.8%
5. *Proportional method:*
   $N = 10$, average 21.4%, range 2.9% to 34.5%

The amount of usable meat an animal could have provided to the prehistoric diet is usually calculated as a percentage of the body weight of an animal. Usable meat is defined as the weight of the animal excluding the weight of the skin, skeleton, and viscera. Clearly, this is an average approximation, as we know that in some cases parts of the viscera and even the hide are eaten, or to the other extreme in which only the animal's tongue was eaten. Estimates of usable meat weight for mammals average 65.5% of the total body weight. The percentage of usable meat in fish may be higher (usable meat in chondrichthians is on the average 86%; in teleosts it is 84%), and turtles may be lower (average usable meat 41%). The percentage used for calculating usable meat is most critical when animals, such as mammals, turtles, and fishes, with very different amounts of meat are compared.

An alternative method of estimating meat yields is by establishing a correlation between a dimension or between skeletal weight and meat weight or soft-tissue weight of the animal rather than the animal's total biomass weight, which has been used in the allometric formulas presented in Table 7.2.

The five methods described provide two different types of information. One type of information assumes that the meat used was only that adhering to the bones that were identified in the sample. The other assumes that the meat yielded by each individual animal represented, even if only by a fragment, was entirely consumed. An ethnographic analogy may clarify these two approaches.

From ethnographic evidence, we know that, generally, when large animals are hunted, the carcass is cut into portions, which are distributed according to particular social regulations among the members of the community. What one would expect to find in the refuse of any one household unit would be the enduring remains of the smaller animals that were entirely used by that family, as well as the family's share of larger animals caught by several members of the community. The family's share of the community hunt would be an estimate of the body weight that would adhere to the bone which has survived in excavated refuse. This community-hunt share estimation could be determined by any of the three methods that base body-weight estimates on correlations with the skeletal weight, namely the percentage, scaling (skeletal mass allometry), and proportion methods. Estimates of the family-unit consumption are the product of the minimum number of individuals in the sample and their live weight estimates by using either the White or scaling (dimensional allometry) methods.

These two approaches differ in the procedure for estimation of animal biomass, and in their results. The family-unit consumption estimation quite clearly results in higher biomass values, as the estimate is a product of animal weight and numbers of individuals which may only be represented by a tooth or sliver of bone. The community-hunt share approach based directly on the archeological finds, that is, the weight of skeletal fragments, is, on the other hand, more conservative. One would expect that in some sites meat was obtained by a combination of the family-unit consumption of entire animals and share of part of a large animal resulting from a community hunt. A similar distinction may be made in sites where a market system was in operation. Under such circumstances, one might expect a family to eat an entire chicken or mullet but only the ham of a pig or loin of a cow. If the family's share of the community hunt was always the same cut of meat, or if the housewife purchased only hams, one might be able to distinguish the result of a shared carcass or market purchase by the repeated representation of that species by one or a few skeletal elements. Only under rare circumstances would the share be consistently one cut so that a community-hunt share could be identified.

Whichever approach is taken, one must assume that meat constituted only part of the diet. The plant contribution to the diet is difficult to assess. It is possible with chemical analysis of bone to establish the relative proportion of plant and animal food in the diet (Chapter 5). Ethnographic analogy may also be applied, providing a guide to the relative use of plants and animal food by people of various cultures and living in different geographic settings. Clearly, in the reconstruction of a prehistoric way of life, any such analogy will be speculative, and at best provide an educated guess of the importance of meat in the diet and hunting and fishing as a subsistence activity. Although such a reconstruction must be based on incomplete knowledge and a number of assumptions must be made, we think a range of likely possibilities can justifiably be proposed.

The application of some of these methods to an actual faunal sample may be the best way to illustrate the range of results that may be achieved (Table 7.4). We have purposely chosen a faunal sample of very few different species to simplify the illustration. Such a sample is from the La Chimba site (section 3, level 4) excavated by Alan Osborn in the northern highlands of Ecuador. The site lies at an elevation of 3160 m and was occupied around A.D. 760. This fauna is composed of rabbit (*Sylvilagus brasiliensis*) and three species of deer: white-tailed deer (*Odocoileus virginianus*), a medium-sized deer, probably a brocket (*Mazama* sp.), and a dwarf deer (*Pudu mephistopheles*).

To approximate the biomass resulting from what is here called the family-unit consumption, we have applied the scaling (dimensional) method to the remains in the La Chimba sample. The sample chosen consisted of at least 15 rabbits. The combined estimated body weights of the rabbits is 9098 gm. The deer represented in the sample include 4 adult and 1 juvenile

TABLE 7.4.
Reconstruction of the Relative Importance of Rabbit and Deer in the Diet of the La Chimba People.

	Rabbit	Deer
Family-unit consumption calculations		
Minimum number of individuals	15	7
Percentage of MNI	68	32
Estimated weight	9098 ± 2420	184,349 ± 49,037
Scaling (dimensional) percentage		
contribution	4.7 (2.8–7.9)	95.3 (92.2–97.2)
Share of community hunt calculations		
Sample bone weight	183	2992
Percentage of bone weight	5.8	94.2
Estimated weight		
scaling (skeletal mass)	3144 ± 377	53,346 ± 6,402
percentage contribution	5.6 (4.4–7.0)	94.4 (93.0–95.6)
Estimated weight		
percentage method	2440 ± 756	39,893 ± 12,367
percentage contribution	5.8 (3.1–10.4)	94.2 (89.6–96.9)
Estimated weight		
proportion method	5558 ± 1167	52,673 ± 11,061
percentage contribution	9.5 (6.5–13.9)	90.5 (86.1–93.6)
Calories per 100 gm portion[a]	125	126
Protein grams per 100 gm portion	21	21
Grams of meat[b]	22	200
Calories[b]	30	252
Grams of protein[b]	4.6	42

[a] Watt and Merrill 1963.
[b] Assuming meat contributed 15% of the calories in a 2000 calorie per day diet.

white-tailed deer, 1 brocket, and 1 Pudu. The combined estimated weight of these animals is 184,349 gm. In terms of biomass, deer contribute 95.3% and rabbit 4.7% to the catch of the family-unit consumption, as reflected in this sample.

Estimation of the community-hunt share is based on the weight of bone in the sample. Bone identified as rabbit weighs 183 gm, and identified deer remains weigh 2992 gm. By using the scaling method, which correlates body weight with skeletal weight, the estimated deer weight is 53,346 gm and rabbit weight is 3144 gm. The percentage method, which gave a low estimate for one test animal, results in an estimate for deer of 39,893 gm and rabbit 2440 gm. Using proportion as a guide, the weight estimate of deer is 52,673 gm and rabbit 5558 gm. By any of these methods, deer contribute 91–94% of the biomass, and rabbit contribute 6–10%.

The results of both the approaches, community-hunt and family-unit consumption, are very close in terms of the percentage contribution of rabbits and deer, but differ markedly in the estimates of the biomass that the bones in this sample represent. This may be interpreted as an indication that hunting was conducted by the family unit, and larger animals were not distributed among the community. The discrepancies between the biomass estimates may simply reflect destruction of bone. The differences in the biomass estimates calculated by the scaling methods would suggest that only about one-third of the supporting tissue of the computed minimum number of individuals was preserved.

To range further into speculation, one can compute the caloric or protein contribution of deer and rabbit, assuming a 2000 calorie daily diet comprised 15% of meat (Table 7.4). The methods previously described can then serve as a guide to the relative use of the animal species found. If the assumption that the diet of the inhabitants provided 2000 calories of which 15% was meat is valid, then perhaps the proposed calculations are tenable. Accepting these assumptions tentatively, deer provided 200 gm of meat of which 42 gm was protein and 252 calories, and rabbit provided 22 gm of which 4.6 gm was protein and 30 calories to the average daily diet at La Chimba. For those less accustomed to metric measurements this combined weight of meat is one-half pound of meat a day. Minimum daily requirement of protein is generally based on 1 gram of protein daily for each kilogram of body weight. Thus a person weighing 50 kg (110 pounds) would require 50 gm of protein per day. These allowances are considered to apply to persons normally vigorous and living in Western civilization and in temperate climates. It is quite possible that the people living at La Chimba around A.D. 700 flourished on somewhat less than the recommended dietary allowance of protein. By our calculations, the average daily protein intake was 47 gm which is within reasonable limits.

A comparison between primary and secondary data indicates that estimates of minimum numbers of individuals are similar to the number of fragments and that estimates of biomass are similar to bone weight. As indicated earlier, this may not always be true, particularly when a faunal sample includes species with very different numbers of skeletal elements. In such a sample the number of skeletal fragments and estimate of minimum numbers of individuals may differ widely and the value of making these estimates is to arrive at an approximation of the relative abundance of each of the species represented.

INVERTEBRATE REMAINS

A great array of invertebrate animals are used for food. The most familiar are the molluscs, which include a large variety of clams, oysters, mussels, snails, and conchs, and the crustaceans, a class of the arthropods that include shrimp, crabs, crayfish, and lobsters. Less familiar to the Western diet, but important in many aboriginal diets, are insects that belong to another class of the arthropods. These animals are widely distributed throughout the world. The most easily harvested crustaceans and molluscs abound in coastal waters, particularly in the intertidal zone, as well as in estuarine and fresh water. Insects are abundant in both aquatic and land habitats.

Most of the species of insects that are known to be eaten intentionally are gregarious (Bodenheimer 1951). Masses of water boatmen (Corixidae) eggs that were blown up in windrows at the edge of lakes were gathered by the Aztecs for food. The Yukpa Indians of eastern Colombia, for example, use at least 25 species of insects as a regular food source (Ruddle 1973). Congregations of developing beetle larvae (probably wood-boring beetles of the family Cerambycidae subfamily Prioninae and weavels of the family Curculionidae tribe Rynchophorini) in palm tree trunks form a focal point to the subsistence of some South American tribes (Clastres 1972, Roth 1916–1917/1970). The Indians prepare palm tree trunks to attract these beetles which lay eggs in the wood. The people then return to the logs when the larvae are the right size to eat. This is a resource that is manipulated by people who know the life history and requirements of the insects in the environment. Another insect that is nurtured in a comparable fashion is the bee. A myriad of different species of this social insect, including the tropical species of stingless bees, are used (Schwarz 1948). The products of bees, larvae and honey, are greatly esteemed and nutritious foods, and are eagerly sought.

The unintentionally consumed insects may also have an impact on human nutrition. Insects, both adults and larvae, are ubiquitous in food storage, as well as being quick to feed on ripe nuts, fruits, and fresh leaves. When these infested foods are eaten quite a lot of insect protein may also be consumed. United States government agencies limit the permissible amount of such inclusions that may be sold in foods; however, this is a recent restriction. In the absence of these restrictions, it may be assumed that insect contamination of foods is a common occurrence. Many species of insects are composed of from 35 to 50% protein on a dry weight basis and are also a good source of minerals, particularly phosphorus, calcium, and iodine, which make insects a nutritious additive to grains (DeFoliart 1975).

Invertebrate food sources are generally easy to collect, requiring little complex technology. Most of these animals are slow moving and may simply be gathered. This is particularly true of the molluscs. Many of those most suitable for food live in congregations in the intertidal zone, where they form oyster bars and clam beds. At most, collection of these animals must be timed with the rise and fall of the tides. The Crustacea are generally more mobile, but good catches of crabs and shrimps are possible with nets or basketry traps. A simple circular dip net is used in many areas to catch such varied prey as cray fish, small fishes, frogs, grasshoppers, and dragonflies. Although many invertebrates are easily caught, their abundance or availability may be sharply seasonal, confined to phases of the moon and tides or reproductive cycles of the animal when, for example, certain crabs will emerge from the water or young shrimp penetrate estuaries.

Some of the small molluscs frequently recovered in middens may have been associated with the main catch by virtue of being attached to oyster shells, or the like, or may be small terrestrial gastropods that were attracted to the decomposing litter of trash. These have had little or no impact on the prehistoric diet and therefore will not be discussed further. They may, however, provide important clues about the prehistoric environment, and their value to an understanding of the past is described by Evans (1972) in his book *Land Snails in Archaeology.*

The preservation of the remains of intentionally used invertebrates is not uniform. The shells of molluscs, which may constitute as much as 90% of the total weight of the animal, are particularly durable in alkaline soils. Accumulations of shells in shell middens have endured for millenia, sometimes in thick deposits. A recent report of a shell midden from South Africa is dated at 20,000 to 60,000 years ago, attesting to the long use of this resource (Volman 1978). Remains of Crustacea are by comparison rarely preserved. Occasionally, the thick shell of stone crab claws (*Menippe mercenaria*) are recovered, whereas the delicate exoskeleton of shrimp are almost never found. Desert conditions are optimal for preservation of organic material, and it is in such environments that a fuller range of invertebrate remains can be recovered.

IDENTIFICATION

Identification of the remains of invertebrates is in some respects easier and in other respects harder than the identification of vertebrate remains. With rare exceptions, the hard parts of invertebrates are external, either in the form of a shell as in the molluscs or the exoskeleton of arthropods. External characteristics are those upon which taxonomic distinctions are generally made and, therefore, these are described and illustrated. The difficulty in the identification in these organisms arises from their being less well known taxonomically than vertebrates and, thus, their nomenclature is in a state of flux.

As with all other unidentified material, comparison of the unidentified objects with appropriately identified specimens is essential for accurate identification. The practical alternatives are to make initial and tentative identification of invertebrates using illustrations, descriptions, and keys that are published, and then to verify these identifications with references to specimens in a museum collection or a collection made for the purpose of identifying a particular sample of invertebrate faunal remains. In making a collection of comparative specimens, it must be remembered that proper permits are required for the collection and possession of endangered and threatened animals (see the Appendix). At the time of this writing, many of the North American freshwater mussels are on the endangered list. If specimens in the faunal sample are entire and unbroken, it may be possible to identify them with sufficient confidence that they in turn may be used as comparative specimens for the fragmentary specimens. These identifications will then form the basis for a quantitative analysis of the relative contribution of the identified organisms to the prehistoric diet.

The following references may help in making identifications.

Abbott, R. T.
  1974 *American seashells* (2nd ed.). New York: Van Nostrand Reinhold.
Andrews, Jean
  1971 *Sea shells of the Texas coast.* Austin: Univ. Texas Press.
Burch, J. B.
  1975 *Freshwater Unionacean clams (Mollusca: Pelecypoda) of North America.* Hamburg, Michigan: Malacological Publications.
Crowder, William
  1959 *Seashore life between the tides.* [*Atlantic Coast*]. New York: Dover.
Emerson, W. K., and M. K. Jacobson
  1976 *The American Museum of Natural History guide to shells: Land, freshwater, and marine, from Nova Scotia to Florida.* New York: Knopf.
Felder, Darryl L.
  1973 *An annotated key to crabs and lobsters (Decapoda, Reptantia) from coastal waters of the Northwestern Gulf of Mexico.* Center for Wetland Resources, Louisiana State University, Baton Rouge, Publication No. LSU-SG-73-02.
Gosner, Kenneth L.
  1971 *Guide to identification of marine and estuarine invertebrates. Cape Hatteras to the Bay of Fundy.* New York: Wiley.
Keen, A. Myra
  1971 *Sea shells of tropical West America. Marine mollusks from Baja California to Peru* (2nd ed.). Berkeley: Stanford Univ. Press.
Klots, Elsie B.
  1966 *The new field book of freshwater life.* New York: Putnam.
Miner, R. W.
  1950 *Field book of seashore life.* New York: Putnam.
Morris, P. A.
  1966 *A field guide to shells of the Pacific Coast and Hawaii.* Boston: Houghton Mifflin.
Pennak, R. W.
  1953 *Freshwater invertebrates of the United States.* New York: Ronald Press.
Ricketts, E. F., and J. Calvin
  1952 *Between Pacific tides* (3rd ed., revised by J. W. Hedgpeth). Berkeley: Stanford Univ. Press.
Warmke, G. L., and R. T. Abbott
  1961 *Caribbean seashells.* Wynnewood, Pennsylvania: Livingston Press.

QUANTIFICATION

In the face of such disparate preservation as the inedible parts of shrimp and oyster, as well as deer and squash, how can one assess their relative contribution to the diet? In the absence of archeological data (i.e., the identifiable organic remains which were either not disposed of at the site or not preserved or recovered), little can be said about the use of an unidentified resource. In partial contradiction to this, new methods are being developed by which the consumption of certain foods is implied by the composition of human bone (see Chapter 5). Such techniques still have limited application, and, therefore, most subsistence information is derived from the identified organic remains that are recovered from archeological sites. Since various foods differ so greatly in their inedible portions, these differences must be taken into account in assessing the contribution of each food to the diet.

Shell mounds are often large and conspicuous features of the landscape, giving the impression of sumptuous shellfish feasting. As has been frequently observed, "the shells so apparent in a shell midden do not have to indicate primary dependence on molluscs for food since small quanitities of less visible components may indicate food resources of even greater importance to the inhabitants of the site [Meigham 1969:420]." Two methods are most effectively used to assess the potential magnitude of the importance of shellfish to the diet. These are correlations between the edible portion and the weight of the shell of each species in the sample. The California shell mounds have provided much of the raw data used in grappling with this problem of evaluating the dietary contribution of shellfish.

One of the earliest attempts to gain a measure of the relative importance of shellfish was a calculation of the volume of shells in a midden (Nelson 1909, 1910). This method was found to be less accurate than a computation of the weight of various components in the archeological sample (Cook 1946; Gifford 1916; Greengo 1951). Shell weights and dimensions are the data on which estimates of meat weight and calories are based in a number of studies that attempt to evaluate the dietary contribution of molluscs (Parmalee and Klippel 1974; Shawcross 1967, 1972). One method takes into account the total weight of the remains in each excavation unit and the proportion of these remains that are shell, the average proportion of shell to meat, the observed loss in weight of shell in the deposit through leaching, the calories per 100 gm, and the percentage of error in each step (Shawcross 1967, 1972).

Another method that aims at the same results approaches the problem of determining an estimate of shellfish meat weight from linear dimensions of the shell or weight of the shell by a regression analysis (Parmalee and Klippel 1974). These regression analyses were made using data on the length, width, height, and weight of the shells of 39 species of North American freshwater mussels. These regression formulas are used to estimate the amount of meat that could have been derived from the shells recovered in an excavated sample; caloric and other food values are extracted from tables in *Compositions of Foods* (Watt and Merrill 1963). The margin of error, introduced at each step in calculation of estimates of caloric contribution of the constituents of a diet as well as the population that could be supported, must be considered.

Ethnographic study of the rate of midden accumulation, selection of shellfish from the available molluscan fauna, size of shellfish meals consumed, and calculations of coastal productivity provide some of the insight needed for the interpretation of prehistoric shell middens (Bailey 1975; Voigt 1975). Ethnographic study of a family and the shellfish they collected and ate as well as the shell midden that this family had accumulated over 46 years provided quantitative data on the rate of consumption and on resource selection which begin to make it possible to suggest norms or ranges for the accumulation and composition of prehistoric shell middens in the same region of South Africa (Voigt 1975). A different approach to a similar problem of interpretation was taken by calculating the caloric yield of the oyster and fishes represented in an Australian shell midden and extrapolating from this how many people could have been supported at this site (Bailey 1975).

The recurring questions that these and other studies pose are the length of the occupation, either from start to the end of the accumulation or the season of each year that the site was occupied, the number of people occupying the site, and the ways in which the shellfish portion of the diet was supplemented. A technique has been developed to help answer one of these questions, namely, that of the season of occupation of the midden site. The basis of this method is the effect of temperature on the variation in the proportion of stable isotopes of oxygen (^{16}O, ^{17}O, and ^{18}O) in calcium carbonate. "The reason is that in the calcification process the distribution of oxygen atoms between host water and the crystal lattice is not quite random: there is a very small isotopic discrimination, and this is temperature dependent (Shackleton 1973:133)." With careful choice of a mollusc that lives in the sea (avoiding the temperature fluctuations of tide pools or sand), that deposit carbonate throughout the year, and that have a growth rate sufficiently great to allow sampling of discrete increments of growth samples of the shell edge may be taken for analysis of the isotope composition. The isotope composition of the edge of the shell which is that laid down just prior to death can be compared to the isotopic composition of shell deposited in previous seasons. This method of determining seasonality in the use of molluscs was applied to a study of the limpets (*Patella tabularis*) from the Nelson Bay cave deposit in South Africa (Shackleton 1973). The specimens from the midden consistently pointed to a winter occupation.

Seasonal consumption of molluscs may be timed to augment the diet when other sources of protein are scarce or to coincide with increased availability or nutritional quality of the molluscs. The nutritional components of a number of foods have been extensively studied, compared, and presented in tables by Watt and Merrill (1963). These may be used to gain an understanding of the contribution of different foods to a diet. They show, for example, that molluscs provide relatively fewer calories, less protein, and more calcium per unit weight than the meat of vertebrates, although this may vary a great deal with the season the molluscs were collected or the stage in their development. This may reveal the complimentarity of some combinations of foods, although such balance in the diet is usually the subtle combination of amino acids.

The interaction of foods is complex and what often appear to be minor changes in the preparation or combination of foods can have profound effects on the diet. The use of lime in the preparation of corn is one example of these that was discussed earlier (p. 66). Mollusc shells are a source of lime for this process. Lime is also used in combination with coca to help extract the alkaloid which is the active ingredient that has an impact on the diet of the user (Burchard 1975). Lime used with coca may be shell but is more often plants with a high calcium content such as quinoa (Gade 1975). Lime containers are illustrated in the fine-line drawing in Mochica art of two individuals chewing coca with lime that is dipped from the gourd container with a spatula (Figure 7.6). Almost identical gourds are used for the same purpose in parts of South America today (Donnan 1976).

This discussion of invertebrate use has emphasized the use of molluscs. This emphasis is not based as much on their importance to the prehistoric diet as their prominance in the prehistoric record. Many invertebrates may

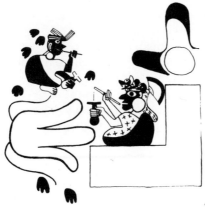

Figure 7-6. A fine line drawing from Mochica art of two individuals using lime along with chewing coca leaves to release the active ingredients in coca (reprinted from *Moche art and iconography* by permission of the author Christopher B. Donnan 1976:95).

have played an equal or even larger role in the prehistoric diet, but this is often hard to document. Remains of the more fragile arthropods and soft bodied invertebrates are found only under unusual conditions of preservation. Evidence of their consumption may be documented in analysis of coprolites, fossilized feces (Chapter 7, p. 151). Even without concrete evidence for a variety of invertebrates in the diet, the possibility of their importance must be considered.

PLANT REMAINS

Of all organic remains, plants are the most fragile and require the most careful techniques in recovering them from archeological sites. Certain plant parts are more durable and thus more frequently recovered. Those parts that have implications to the prehistoric diet are seeds, more precisely disseminules, and pollen. Seeds are rich in nutrients and, therefore, were widely sought for food. As a matter of fact, seeds, such as wheat, barley, rice, and corn, are the staple of most diets based on domestic plants (Heiser 1973). Pollen is produced in even greater quantities than seeds and has an outer coat or exine, which is more durable than the seed coat of seeds. The presence of pollens in an archeological site often results from the dispersal of pollens from flowering plants by wind and thus does not usually reflect the remnants of plants eaten.

Propagative parts of plants, such as seeds, are enclosed in a seed coat and often also by hard woody pericarps or cases that contribute to their frequent preservation. These include what botanists distinguish as caryopses, such as kernels of corn; and grains of grasses, such as wheat; nuts, such as acorn and hickory; stones within the fruits of cherries; and pips or seeds of grapes. Sometimes the fleshy fruit surrounding the seed is eaten, as in the case of pumpkin, squash, and grapes; other times, the seed itself is eaten, as in acorns, corn, beans, pumpkins, and squash.

The environmental conditions favoring preservation are the dry conditions found in deserts or caves or the waterlogged anaerobic conditions of bogs. It is for these reasons that our fullest knowledge of prehistoric plant use in the Western Hemisphere comes from the desert coast of Peru (Towle 1961), Salts and Mammoth Caves in Kentucky (Watson and Yarnell 1966; Watson 1974), rock shelters in the arid Tehuacan Valley (Byers 1967), and

Figure 7-7. Graphs showing changes in dimensions due to carbonization of hulled barley grains (*Hordeum vulgare*) (reprinted by permission of Columbia University Press from *Paleoethnobotany* by Jane M. Renfrew 1973:11). Table comparing the dimensions of prehistoric cereal grains with those of their modern counterparts. Prehistoric cereal grains may differ in size from their exact counterparts of the present day, even when these are also carbonized. (Table reprinted by permission of Columbia Univ. Press from Palaeoethnobotany by Jane M. Renfrew 1973:13.)

some of the sites in the desert Southwest (Bohrer and Adams 1977). The most famous find of waterlogged material is that of the Danish bog corpses in which the food contents of the digestive tract could be identified, giving the most direct evidence of the diet (Helbaek 1954).

The preservation of plant parts is enhanced by carbonization when the climate is too wet for dry preservation. The carbonization of seeds may not alter the surface details of the seed but may change its size and proportions. Experiments were done by Jane Renfrew (1973:9–15) in which she compared several dimensions of carbonized and uncarbonized grains of wheat, barley, oats, and rye (Figure 7.7). These distortions in size and proportions must be considered in making identifications of carbonized grains by comparison with modern fresh grains.

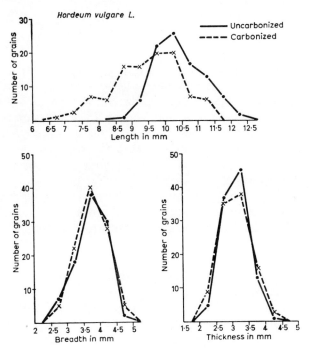

Comparing the Dimensions of Prehistoric Cereal Grains with Those of Their Modern Counterparts

	Length	Breadth	Thickness
	mm	mm	mm
Hordeum vulgare—hulled six-row barley			
prehistoric, carbonized	5.3	3.1	2.5
modern, fresh	7.81	3.55	2.68
modern, carbonized	7.2	3.94	3.11

Another type of evidence for plant use is the impression of plant parts in the clay of pottery, bricks, tabby, or adobe. In the manufacture of these materials, plants may be intentionally or accidentally incorporated and the impression of these plants preserved in the dry or fired clay. These impressions are often accurate images of the plant parts. They may, in fact, incorporate the silica skeletons of the grasses and grains making the impressions. These silica skeletons are the remnants of silica in the interstices between the cellulose cell walls deposited during the growth of the plant. Therefore, these fragile structures accurately reflect the detailed cellular anatomy of the plants (Dimbleby 1967:134–315; Renfrew 1973:16–17). As with the distortions in the size and shape of the charred plant parts, these impressions will be smaller than the plants that made them due to shrinkage during the drying and firing of the clay.

There are well known examples of plant impressions used for decorative motifs on pottery. Those related to food items are the cob-marked pottery of the southeastern United States. The cob-marked pottery was impressed with corn cobs, a plant crop grown presumably for consumption. Oval depressions in some Valdivia period (around 2000 B.C.) pots from the coast of Ecuador are interpreted as being impressions of corn kernels (Zevallos, Galinat, Lathrap, Levy, Marcos, and Klumpp 1977). This evidence is further supported by the identification of corn or maize opal phytoliths in soils associated with archeological soils of that formative period (Pearsall 1978). A further piece of evidence is found in a dog burial also associated with this site in which the ratio of the isotopes of carbon-12 and carbon-13 in the dog's bone collagen (see p. 76) indicates that this domestic animal had a diet composed of 63.5% corn (Burleigh and Brothwell 1978). These combined lines of evidence convincingly support the conclusion of a corn agricultural system in formative times on the coast of Ecuador, with its attendant implications to the diet.

Other types of plant parts that are encountered are the woody portions of the plants associated with the edible parts. Corn cobs are frequently reported and are of prime interest in tracing the domestication of this plant and the spread of corn agriculture. Some of the oldest and most primitive cobs, only three quarters of an inch long, were excavated from the Tehuacan Valley, Mexico (Byers 1967). These document the use of corn as early as 5000 B.C. Associated with these finds of corn cobs are quids of chewed corn stalks and husks as well as quids of agave leaves and mesquite. Pods of beans, mesquite, acacia, and pochote were also encountered in the Tehuacan Valley caves.

The preservation of plant remains in the caves in the arid Tehuacan Valley is remarkable. Identified were the remains of well over 50 species associated with archeological strata extending over a time span of over 8000 years. Under less favorable conditions fewer plant remains are preserved; however "Helbaek, with his wide experience of archaeological sites in the Near East, has averred that in his opinion every site holds some botanical evidence; we must prepare ourselves to ensure that it is not overlooked as it has so often been in the past [Dimbleby 1967:149]."

Microscopic remains of plants such as pollen and phytoliths require special techniques for extraction from the soil and a different approach to interpretation. They will be discussed in greater detail in the following section.

IDENTIFICATION

The method of identification of fragmentary plant remains follows a, by now, familiar sequence. The details are, of course, specific to the taxonomic group. As with the identification of vertebrates and invertebrates, the key characteristics vary from one group to another, and the degree of difference separating species is no more uniform in plants than in animals. Key characteristics are shape, size, proportions and details of sculpturing, pores, hairs, and the plant structure as they can be seen in the remains. Bohrer and Adams (1977), in their very useful manual on ethnobotanical techniques, advocate an approach to the identification of botanical remains that is followed here. The basic steps in the procedure are: (*a*) determine order or family affiliation of the unknown plant; (*b*) compare it with the species of the flora in the region of the site, particularly those plants with known ethnobotanical use and those plants occupying disturbed habitats; (*c*) compare it with descriptions and illustrations in a botanical manual, for example, a seed identification manual; and (*d*) verify initial identification by comparison of the unknown sample with vouchered or comparative specimens.

To make a project of identification of plant remains manageable, the list of potential plants must be narrowed down. This can be done in several ways. First, a list of the plants native to the vegetation in the area of the site would be combined with a list of plants that might have been cultivated. This combined list would then form the basic checklist of species to investigate—keep in mind that the vegetation around the site may have been different when it was occupied, and adjustments in the floral lists might have to be made to include extrapated species. This list can be narrowed down by eliminating poisonous and inedible species. Here again, care must be exercised as inedibility is in part a subjective value, and some poisonous plants can be rendered harmless by the method of preparation. Certain plants or parts of plants are, however, never eaten, because they are too toxic or cannot be digested by human beings. The list can be further refined by isolating for more detailed study those plants that are known to have been used.

With the scope of the plant species thus narrowed down, the unknown plant remains can be identified as to their affiliation with the larger taxonomic units, order and family. Such a sorting can be done with the help of articles and books, such as *Seed Collecting and Identification* by Gunn (1972) and *Seeds and Fruits of Plants of Eastern Canada and Northeastern United States* by Montgomery (1977). For determination of generic characteristics more detailed and specific guides must be consulted.

As with the identification of other biological remains, unknown material must be compared with securely identified voucher specimens for an accurate identification to the generic or specific level. A seed collection may already be established in a local or regional herbarium. In particularly difficult cases of identification, it may be possible, by prior arrangement, to use such a facility or to seek the help of the specialists employed. The other alternative is to start a seed collection for a specific research problem.

In starting such a collection, seeds should be accompanied by herbarium specimens of the whole plants so the identification of the seeds can be verified (Gunn 1972; Smith 1971).

QUANTIFICATION

In the interpretation of prehistoric consumption of plants based on the recovery and identification of plant remains, the biases introduced by poor preservation must be considered. Just as oysters and shrimp differ in the durability and amount of their hard and inedible parts, and thus in their preservation in an archeological site, so does the preservation of beans and corn differ compared with manioc and potatoes. Another source of bias in a comparison between the remains of plant and animal foods is that the remains of animal sources of food are the inedible skeletal or exoskeletal parts, whereas the remains of plant foods are often the food itself in the form of charred kernels of corn or carbonized marsh-elder seeds.

With these biases in mind, one must be cautious in interpreting the contribution of different plants to the diet based solely on recovered plant remains. The botanical remains may be enumerated so that information about the nature and identification of each specimen and its location in the site is included in the tabulation. New techniques, such as trace mineral analysis and carbon isotope studies (see Chapter 5), can provide important support for the accuracy with which the recovered botanical remains reflect the plants that were consumed.

The evaluation of the botanical remains as evidences of "first-line foods" or intensively harvested plants will take into account the nutritional value of the food, the ease with which it may be stored, the methods by which it may be harvested, and its relative abundance in the site (Asch, Ford, and Asch 1972). Sources for these types of information are scattered. The nutritional values as well as the inedible portion of many foods are presented in the handbook on *Composition of Foods* (Watt and Merrill 1963). Among the most nutritionally valuable and frequently encountered plant remains in temperate regions are nuts. Estimations of the numbers of whole nuts in a portion of a site, based on their charred fragmentary remains, must take into account the loss of weight in the shell as a result of charring. In estimating the importance of hickory nuts at the Koster site in Illinois, an experiment was performed to determine the average loss in weight of the nutshells after carbonization. The average shell weight of one nut decreased from 1.67 gm to .81 gm after carbonization (Asch *et al.* 1972). Thus, assuming that all parts of the nutshell were recovered and they were all carbonized equally, 0.81 gm of nutshell fragments is equivalent to one nut, and the 1053 gm of nutshells in the flotation sample is estimated to represent the remains of 1300 whole nuts. Using comparable methods, the proportions of different nut remains recovered in the flotation samples of a site can reflect the differential use of these forest products. This, in turn, must be related to the past vegetation in the area surrounding the site and the nut-bearing regime of the trees.

Remains of nuts from five different kinds of trees were identified from the Koster Site (Asch *et al.* 1972). These nuts come from trees that bear fruit at different seasons, with hazelnuts ripe in August and September before the other nuts ripen. Nut trees do not bear a good crop every year but may produce nuts every 2 or 3 years or as seldom as 5 or more years. A poor crop of nuts from one kind of tree may be offset by a good crop from another kind, making a dependence on a variety of nuts a more secure sort of existence (Dimbleby 1967:35–37). Hazelnuts bear best in full sunlight, although they are a deciduous forest tree. This preference was probably learned by people depending on hazelnuts and may have spurred selective clearing of the forests (Dimbleby 1967). Such ecological information about plants must be considered in an evaluation of their past use.

It may be taken as axiomatic that plants were important to all but the most specialized diets. Furthermore, recovered and identified plant remains are but a scant trace of the plant constituents of the prehistoric diet. With improved recovery techniques and increased concern about the types of information plant remains may provide, the evidences for the kinds and relative quantities of plants consumed is mounting. The evidences of plant remains are now possible to augment by studies of trace minerals in human bone (Chapter 5) and by analysis of coprolites (Chapter 7, p. 151).

MICROSCOPIC BIOLOGICAL REMAINS

Because of their size, microscopic and small macroscopic organic remains require special techniques for recovery and study. Small animal remains include skeletal fragments, mainly of small vertebrates, such as: mice; song birds; frogs; lizards; herrings and other small fishes; chitinous remains of insects; eggs of parasites; hair; feathers; and scales. Microscopic botanical remains include pollen, spores, phytoliths, stellate hairs, and other epidermal fragments. Many of these may be recovered from midden material by special methods. Both plant and animal remains may also be extracted from coprolites. Plant remains may be extracted from soil samples taken at the site, but soil samples, though valuable for environmental reconstruction, have no necessary connection with prehistoric diets. Flotation sampling is the means by which most botanical remains are recovered. Normally, float samples will also include remains of animals, both small fragments of larger animals and remains of small-sized species used at the site, as well as those accidentally incorporated in the midden. Burrowers and other animals of accidental or post-depositional occurrence were discussed in the previous sections.

The most direct evidence of the foods consumed is their remains in coprolites. These objects may contain undigested remnants of food that had a direct impact on the diet. They may also contain evidence of parasites, implying a drain on the nutrition of the individual. Of less direct implication to the diet are the pollen and phytoliths extracted from the soils of the archeological site. These may reflect plants used at the site, but, more commonly, are a sample of the natural or disturbed vegetation in its vicinity.

Identification of small or microscopic remains requires comparison with specimens of known identity, as was described for macroscopic remains. Sometimes this is easy, as hair must come from mammals and feathers from birds. The task of identifying these may be simplified if they belong to species already identified from larger remains. However, species represented solely by microscopic remains should be expected, and their identification should proceed by a process of elimination.

SPECIAL TECHNIQUES FOR RECOVERY AND INTERPRETATION OF MICROSCOPIC REMAINS

SIEVING

Sieving of archeological materials was discussed earlier (p. 7), but, because of the importance of sieving in the recovery of organic remains, it will be reviewed again here. The finest screen gauges, of approximately window screen size (1.4 mm), must be used to recover small vertebrate remains and plant seeds. Under certain very arid conditions the midden matrix can be sieved through the screen dry. Often, however, water must be used to wash the soil through the screen. Once wet, the organic material must be carefully and slowly dried. Too rapid shrinking and swelling that accompanies wetting and drying can make fragile remains break into smaller and even less easily identifiable pieces.

FLOTATION

The underlying principle of flotation techniques is that organic material is lighter (has a lower specific gravity) than inorganic material. Thus, a means of separating the organic from the inorganic soils is by floating the organic remains on the surface of water, while heavier particles sink. A number of elaborate devices have been designed, and additives to the solution have been tested that aid in the flotation and separation of the organic material (Struever 1968; Jarman, Legge, and Charles 1972; Renfrew, Monk, and Murphy 1975). Perhaps the simplest method was described to the Real Mesoamerican Archeologists and is quoted here as follows:

> Gray ash and black ash are good bets for flotation samples; so is ashy brown earth with visible charcoal flecks. White ash is not so good, because the burning is too complete and the oxidation too strong to promote carbonization. Take as big a sample as you can. A 2-kilo bag is good, but a 5-gallon wicker basket lined with newspaper is better. Let the sample dry for a week, very slowly, in the shade; if it dries in the sun, the seed coat shrinks faster than the inner seed, and it cracks.

> Now fill a plastic washtub with water, and add a couple of teaspoons of sodium silicate ("water glass") to each liter of water. The silicate acts as a deflocculant, to disperse the clay and bring the charcoal to the surface clean. Pour in some cupfuls of dirt from the sample, stir, and when you think all the carbon is floating, pour it off into a screen before it starts to waterlog. Be generous with the water, and pour only carbon, not mud, into your screen. When the screen is full, let it dry for a day in the shade, slowly. And there are carbonized seeds.

> Remember, a 5-mm mesh will only stop avocado pits and corncob fragments. A 1.5-mm mesh will stop chile pepper seeds, but if you want the chenopods, amaranths, and smaller field weeds, you have to turn to carburetor mesh [From K. V. Flannery, *The early Mesoamerican village,* © 1976 by Academic Press, New York, pp. 104–105].

DIETARY IMPORTANCE

The dietary impact of the organisms represented by very small remains must be carefully evaluated, just as the larger animals must be evaluated in the reconstruction of a prehistoric diet. Animals in small packages, such as oysters, herrings, or sardines, may have an important impact on the diet if they are eaten in large quantities. Therefore, the small size of the individual does not necessarily mean the item is unimportant. On the other hand, small organisms found in middens may not have been used at all. Many kinds of scavenging animals are attracted to refuse or to stored food. Granary pests, such as mice and insects, are well known; in fact few, if any, granaries are free of such uninvited guests. Other animals may welcome the same shelter used by people. Barn owls often inhabit rock shelters and caves also used by people. Owls regurgitate the indigestible parts of their meals in the form of a pellet. These include bones and hair of their animal prey.

It may be difficult to distinguish between the remains of animals used for food by the human inhabitants of the site and those that have been incidentally incorporated in the site. One method employed to indicate these differences is based on the rationale that an animal that died at the place where its remains are found will be represented by its entire skeleton, whereas an animal that was killed at a distance from the site will have a less complete skeleton present. This method was devised by Shotwell (1955, 1958) to distinguish between "proximal and distal communities" as represented by vertebrate remains in alluvium. It was adapted for archeological materials by Thomas (1971).

One aspect of differential transport is called the "Schlepp Effect" by Perkins and Daly (1968). The Schlepp means literally dragging, as applied to dragging an animal carcass home from the kill site. The farther the carcass has to be dragged, and the larger the carcass, the less of the relative heavy, inedible bone portion that will arrive at the site. Consequently, the representation of that species in the zooarcheological record will be poorer.

The relative completeness of the species represented at a site, or part of a site, may be compared by the method presented by Thomas (1971). His "corrected number of specimens per individual" (CSI) takes into account several types of data which will differ according to the site and to the nature of the remains. The information that must be recorded for the site in question is the number of specimens identified for each species or genus, and the minimum number of individuals of each species or genus. Also recorded is an estimate of the expected number of identifiable elements which would include those bones that would be expected to be recovered and those that can be positively identified; thus, this estimate would differ from species to species. The corrected specimens per individual (CSI) is calculated for each species or genus in the assemblage by the formula:

$$CSI = \frac{100 \text{ (number of specimens)}}{\text{(expected number) (MNI)}}$$

expected number = estimated number of identifiable elements per individual

A comparison of the resulting corrected number of specimens per individual in a faunal assemblage may be graphed to illustrate both relative completeness and relative abundance of each species. Such a graph is made on a polar grid, where the size of the wedge indicates the relative abundance of each species (based on numbers of identified specimens), and the height or radius of each wedge reflects relative completeness of each species. The coefficient of relative completeness, B, is obtained by the following formula:

$$B = 5 - \text{Log}_e \ CSI$$

This procedure is illustrated by faunal data from the 2500 B.C. occupation at Pikamachay Cave, a rockshelter in the central Andes of Peru (Table 7.5, 7.6, Fig. 7.8). In this sample, the small cricetine rodents are the most abundantly represented and are represented by the most complete skeletons. They and song birds would make up what Shotwell, in the original formulation of this method, would call the proximal population. As the least obviously "schlepped" elements of the faunas, small animals are here interpreted as being largely incidental to the faunal assemblage of animals used by man. In support of this interpretation are finds of mummified rodents, not included in the diagram, and the absence of burned bones among the small animal remains; many of the bones of larger animals were burned. The interpretation of which animals were used and which are incidental to the site must be decided individually for each kind of animal and for each site. The completeness of skeletal representation is merely one bit of evidence that can be used.

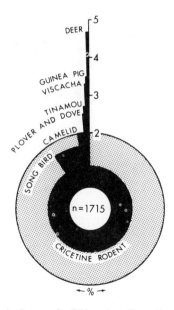

Figure 7-8. Faunal analysis diagram for Pikimachay Cave (Ac 100) in the Ayacucho Valley of Peru. Size of wedge indicates relative frequency. The black portion represents the B value for each species.

TABLE 7.5.

Presentation of Faunal Data from One Cultural Horizon at Pikimachay Cave—Mammal Skeletal Elements[a]

Mammal Skeletal Elements	Llamas and their kin		Deer		Viscacha		Guinea pig		Small rodents	
	Expected	Observed	Expected	Observed	Expected	Observed	Expected	Observed	Expected	Observed
Cranium	1		1		1		1	2	1	110
Mandible	2	4	2		2		2	8	2	391
Teeth	24	1	24		16		16			
Scapula	2	2	2		2		2		2	15
Humerus	2	3	2		2		2		2	154
Radius	2		2		2		2		2	6
Ulna	2	1	2		2		2		2	27
Pelvis	2	4	2		2		2	2	2	198
Femur	2		2		2		2		2	398
Tibia	2	1	2	1	2		2		2	263
Metapodial	4	12	4							
Calcaneum	2	1	2		2	1	2			
Astragalus	2		2		2	1	2			
Phalanx	24		24							
Total number	73	29	73	1	37	2	37	12	17	1562
Minimum number of individuals		2		1		1		7		199
Total weight (gms)		615.7		2.7		1.2		0.44		181.9
Corrected number of specimens per individual (CSI)		19.9		1.4		5.4		4.6		46.2
Coefficient of relative completeness (B)[b]		2.01		4.66		3.31		3.47		1.17
Percentage total number		1.7		0.06		0.1		0.7		91.1

[a]Data used in diagram on Figure 7.8.

[b]$B = 5 - \mathrm{Log}_e / CSI$.

Table 7.6.

Presentation of Faunal Data from One Cultural Horizon at Pikimachay Cave—Bird Skeletal Elements[a]

Bird Skeletal Elements	Plover		Doves		Tinamou		Song Birds	
	Expected	Observed	Expected	Observed	Expected	Observed	Expected	Observed
Cranium	1		1		1		1	7
Sternum	1		1		1		1	
Coracoid	2		2		2		2	3
Humerus	2		2	1	2	1	2	33
Radius	2		2		2		2	
Ulna	2	1	2		2		2	19
Carpometacarpus	2	1	2	1	2		2	7
Pelvis–sacrum	2		2		2		2	1
Femur	2	1	2	.	2	1	2	4
Tibiotarsus	2		2		2		2	14
Tarsometatarsus	2		2	1	2		2	13
Total number	20	3	20	3	20	2	20	101
Minimum number of individuals		1		1		1		18
Total weight (gm)		0.08		0.11		0.07		2.85
Corrected number of specimens per individual (CSI)		15		15		10		28
Coefficient of relative completeness (B)[b]		2.29		2.29		2.7		1.67
Percentage total number		0.2		0.2		0.1		5.9
Total	1715							
Total minimum number of individuals	231							

[a] Data used in diagram on Figure 7.8.

[b] $B = 5 - \text{Log}_e / CSI.$

153

COPROLITE ANALYSIS

Coprolites contain undigested food remains which are direct evidence of foods that were eaten. The remains that can be extracted from coprolites include (a) plant remnants such as seeds, pollen, phytoliths, and other plant parts; (b) remains of animal origin such as bone, feathers, hair, and insect chitin; (c) parasites; and (d) inorganic material. A bibliography to "Analysis of ancient feces" (Wilke and Hall 1975) provides information on the full range of materials recovered and identified from coprolites.

Preparation of these diverse types of remains must be carefully planned for the optimal recovery of all components. The procedure outlined here is described in greater detail by Bryant (1974a) in his paper on "The role of coprolite analysis in archeology." The first step is to accurately determine what animal produced the coprolite. This determination is followed by disaggregation of the coprolite, assisted where necessary by mild chemical treatment, so that its organic constituents can be identified.

Several criteria are used to identify the human origin of coprolites. The shape and size easily differentiates human feces from those of large herbivores. The distinction between human and carnivore feces is less clear. Carnivore feces often have a "hard outer coating of dried intestinal lubricant (Bryant 1974a:4)" by which they can be recognized as different from human feces.

The chemical reaction of the coprolite with the usual disaggregating solvent, .5% trisodium phosphate,[2] provides other indications of the source of the coprolite. The human coprolite turns the trisodium phosphate solution dark brown or black and makes it opaque. As far as is now known, only the coprolites of the coati (Nasua nasua) also turn the solution black and opaque, but dark extractable material, presumably nitrogenous, is to be expected in any fresh feces before weathering fossilization. The coprolites of dogs would be most likely to be confused with those of humans (because of dog's close association with human habitation), but dog feces contain a high proportion of ground bone and are white even when relatively fresh. Dog coprolites are similar to those of other carnivores in yielding a white, pale brown, or yellow color in extraction with trisodium phosphate.

Human coprolites may also be distinguished by their color during disaggregation. The odor of human coprolites is similar to that of their fresh state, whereas that of carnivore coprolites is musty.

A final characteristic that sets human feces apart is directly related to the uniquely omnivorous human diet. The wide range of diverse components found in the human coprolites is rarely seen in coprolites of other animals.

[2]Sold in paint and hardware stores as TSP. Calgon and other U.S. commercial detergents are no longer made of trisodium phosphate.

The criterion of diversity applies to populations, however, and nondiverse individual coprolites are not necessarily nonhuman. Finds of host specific parasites, such as the human pinworm *Enterobius vermicularis*, are the most conclusive evidence that the coprolite is of human origin.

For disaggregation, mechanical breaking of the coprolite may work satisfactorily when the coprolite is dry or mineralized. Chemical disaggregation is, however, preferable so that all of the components may be recovered. The methods described here are those developed by the late Eric O. Callen (1963, 1967) and Vaughn M. Bryant (1974a). The procedure used by them is as follows:

1. Photograph and describe the appearance of each coprolite, give linear measurements and weight.
2. Clean thoroughly to remove any pollen that may be contaminating the surface.
3. The coprolite, or the portion of it to be analyzed, is then covered with a .5% solution of trisodium phosphate and sealed in an airtight container for at least 72 hours; it may be kept in the solution indefinitely without destroying the sample.
4. Once the coprolite has broken down, the color of the liquid, its odor, and the presence of a surface scum should be noted.
5. The disintegrated coprolite specimen is then sieved through clean 20 (841 μ) and 65 (210 μ) mesh brass screens and rinsed with a jet of distilled water.
6. The liquid that passes through the screens may contain pollen grains and opal phytoliths which must be concentrated by centrifuging the liquid portion.
7. The portions of the sample caught in the screens are dried and stored for taxonomic study.

The portions recovered in the screens, and composed of small vertebrate and invertebrate remains, seeds, and various plant tissues, are studied, as are other small and microscopic fragments. Usually under the stereobinocular microscope, the remains are sorted along taxonomic lines; based on the characteristics of each preserved fragment, its identity is narrowed down to family or genus, and then identification is made by comparison with identified modern specimens.

POLLEN EXTRACTION AND IDENTIFICATION

Pollen grains are among the most durable and widely distributed parts of plants. The outer coat or exine of the pollen grain is composed of an extraordinarily resistant organic material (sporo-pollenin), which under the right circumstances can persist for thousands of years; in fact, unchanged spore walls have been found in Paleozoic rocks (Faegri and Iversen 1966). The optimal conditions for the survival of exines are found in continuously wet, organic, and anaerobic depositional environments, like that found in bogs, marshes, or lake bottoms. Deposits of pollen are the result of the production of pollen in astronomical numbers of plants and the subsequent dispersal of this pollen by the wind. Wind-pollinated plants, therefore, dominate most pollen assemblages; species pollinated by animals (insects, birds, bats) produce much less pollen and their heavier, more ornamented grains rarely form significant components of the regional pollen rain.

Pollen associated with archeological sites may have been deposited in a pollen rain or may have come from flowers brought to the site. If contamination can be confidently excluded, pollen extracted from coprolites may be interpreted as having come from flowers or from pollen-dusted vegetable parts that were consumed. The evidence from coprolites is the only direct implication of pollen in the diet. In the more usual applications of palynology, pollen taken in or near an archaeological site may reveal past vegetation, including human modifications of the vegetation, such as forest clearing and agriculture. Ideally, as pollen assemblages vary widely for natural or cultural reasons, or for no ascertainable reason, interpretation of assemblages is best done stratigraphically by comparing sequences within the site with those observed in "standard" sections in nearby lakes or bogs.

The methods of pollen analysis are difficult on several counts. Major among these is that all pollen is microscopic, requiring sophisticated knowledge of microscopy, including electron microscopy, for identification. Another major difficulty stems from the pervasiveness of airborne pollen, requiring quasi-microbiological techniques to avoid contamination, both during sampling at the site and during laboratory preparation.

The techniques for preparing a sample involve concentrating the pollen, removing extraneous matter by physical and chemical means, and preparing a slide of the extracted pollen so that several hundred can be examined microscopically. The exact procedure for achieving this may differ between laboratories. In all laboratories, however, scrupulous cleanliness to avoid contamination must be maintained, and precautions in handling certain dangerous chemicals must be observed. The steps in this procedure are fully described in the *Textbook of Pollen Analysis* by Faegri and Iversen (1966) and will not be repeated here in any detail. Basically, however, after chemical disaggregation, large particles are removed from the sample by straining it through 20 (841 μ) mesh and 65 (210 μ) mesh brass screens, the carbonates from the fraction that passed through the screen are removed by using hydrochloric acid; the silicates are removed by hydrous hydroflouric acid;

and the organic material, other than pollen, is removed (after dehydration in glacial acetic acid) by acetolysis (9 cc acetic anhydride to 1 cc sulfuric acid). Finally, the chemicals are washed out, and the pollen is stained and mounted on a slide. The pollen exines will have to be magnified between 300 and 1000 times for study and usually 200 pollen grains are identified and counted in each sample. Modifications of this basic procedure may be warranted, depending on the nature of the sample.

Pollen is identified in the same way as other material, that is, by comparison with identified material. A pollen herbarium containing specimens of all the plants from the vicinity of the site is an essential reference for pollen identification. Pollen collected for herbarium purposes must be handled as rigorously as the samples to be studied. To make these pollen grains comparable in size and in other characteristics, the interior parts of the grain and the extra-exinous oils must be removed by acetolysis, leaving only the exine to be mounted (in the same mounting medium) on a slide. The techniques for these preparations are also described by Faegri and Iversen (1966). Manuals and keys to pollen types exist, but these are not adequate substitutes for the actual comparison of specimens.

The taxonomic level of pollen identification is generally not to species, as is often possible with seed identification. Usually the genus, sometimes the family, is the lowest taxon that can be accurately reached in pollen identification. Identification to species may sometimes be possible with scanning electron microscope. Even more general levels of taxonomic differentiation can be reached by study of opal phytoliths, the other microscopic plant remnant.

OPAL PHYTOLITH EXTRACTION AND IDENTIFICATION

Most recognizable phytoliths are bodies of opaline silica $(SiO_2 \cdot nH_2O)$ deposited in the cells of plants. Calcium oxalate crystals also occur in many plants, but these are not distinctive in form. Phytoliths occur in many different kinds of plants but are particularly common in grasses. They are present in various plant cells, which may in part explain the differences seen in their morphology. A given plant may have many differently shaped phytoliths, some of which are plain, undifferentiated rods of little taxonomic value, while others are distinctive in shape and proportion and, therefore, more useful taxonomically.

Phytoliths often occur in the same types of deposits in which pollen is found. Like pollen grains, phytoliths are microscopic and range in size from 2 to 1000 μm, though most are between 20 and 200 μm in length. They are also very resistant to decay. Phytoliths are very abundantly incorporated in soil, but in contrast to pollen they are deposited as a result of the decomposition of vegetation. Phytoliths will of course not be found on a slide of pollen from which the silica has been removed by hydrofluoric acid. Because some phytoliths may be airborne, especially after fires or in dry weather, the same care to avoid contamination must be taken in preparing a phytolith slide as is taken with the preparation of pollen.

Phytoliths are extracted from soil by chemical and physical methods. Detailed description of the method is found in a paper by Rovner (1971) entitled "Potential of opal phytoliths for use in paleoecological reconstruction." Briefly, the method involves digestion of the organic material and solution of the carbonates by hydrochloric acid (HCl). This is followed by separation of the heavy soil particles from the lighter phytoliths (specific gravity from 1.5 to 2.3) by floating the phytoliths in a heavy liquid mixture of tetrabromethane and absolute ethyl alcohol with a specific gravity of 2.3. The suspended phytoliths are decanted, washed, dried, and mounted on a microscopic slide. For the preparation of comparative phytoliths from known plants, the organic plant material is digested by any of a number of acids. Chromic acid, nitric acid, and a combination of nitric and perchloric acid have been used (Rovner 1971; Armitage 1975), but perchloric acid is very dangerous and must be used only in a specially designed hood. Heat should not be used to extract phytoliths as temperatures over 100 C will distort the phytoliths. Alternatively, the phytoliths may be exposed by epidermal peels of mature leaf segments (Pearsall 1978).

Phytoliths have not been studied in the detail that pollen has, and, therefore, their limitations for taxonomic use are not fully known. It is clear that they are not as distinctive taxonomically as pollen, and that they are perhaps most useful in distinguishing major groups of grasses.

Phytoliths have been found in a number of different archeological situations. As indicated earlier, they are not destroyed in the digestive tract and may be recovered from coprolites, giving direct evidence of plants that were consumed (Bryant 1974a). Their prevalence in grasses makes them particularly useful in studies of the diets of grazing animals (Armitage 1975). In such studies, phytoliths are recovered from droppings as well as from the surface of teeth of ruminants (Armitage 1975). As phytoliths are remnants of decayed vegetation, they may indicate the former presence of deteriorated thatch, straw bedding, or threshed grain when found in archeological soils (Pearsall 1978).

CHEMICAL RESIDUE

Chemical residues of organic material are a potential source of information about food remains. The most sensitive chemical techniques are required for such analyses. Modern techniques of analytical chemistry are very sophisticated and can be applied to a number of archeological problems. Trace-mineral analysis has already been discussed (see Chapter 5). Elemental analysis of the composition of archeological remains has been applied to material such as pottery and metal (Beck 1974). This has less direct application to nutritional reconstruction than does analysis of food residues.

Food residues include organic substances such as carbohydrates, lipids, and amino acids. These can sometimes be found in cooking pots or storage vessels. In a most interesting example, the contents of a vial excavated from a site in Ethiopia were subjected to amino-acid analysis by ion-exchange chromatography (Von Endt 1977). The amino acids of the residue were compared with those of civet cat protein, leading to the conclusion that the vial contained civet-cat gland exudate originally used in perfume. Although this is of course not a food, similar techniques might be applied to a food residue, providing nutritional data.

Some of the techniques that have been discussed in this section require sophisticated equipment and procedures, such as those involved in the extraction of pollen grains or the analysis of amino acids. Other techniques, such as water screening and flotation, have already become routine in the recovery of archeological remains. The data resulting from these various techniques have different implications to a reconstruction of prehistoric diets. The full potentials of some of these methods are yet to be realized.

Procurement Patterns and 8
Dietary Regimes

The preceding chapters have been devoted to a discussion of methods used to study prehistoric procurement patterns and diets. Some of these methods, such as the search for dental caries among human remains and the identification of animal bones, have become quite standard in archeological research. Other methods, such as strontium analysis and palynology, require complex techniques and are just now being applied to the reconstruction of prehistoric diets. The greatest insight into prehistoric nutrition will be possible as the older techniques become perfected, the newer methods become widely applied, and all of the resulting data are integrated.

The aim of such studies is to more fully understand the range of adaptations of human foodways that ensure the survival of the cultural group. A myriad of challenges are faced in coping with the potentials and limitations of different environments and by the nutritional requirements of the individual. A number of different models and mechanisms have been proposed to help explain ways peoples have coped with such problems as the seasonal abundance and scarcity of food resources, provision of food to concentrations of people, and ways of obtaining a diet with sufficient calories and balanced nutrients.

SEASONAL ABUNDANCE AND
SCARCITY OF FOOD RESOURCES

Change is one of the characteristics of life and the nonliving environment. The annual fluctuations in the availability of resources is a response to seasonal changes in temperature or moisture and the reproductive growth cycle of plants and animals. Superimposed on these cycles are longer fluctuations in the size of yields of the mast crop, or rabbit population density, or the position of the equatorial current. In the face of the complexity of these fluctuations in abundance of organic resources, people must eat on a regular basis.

Not only must people eat regularly, but the cost in terms of energy expenditure of obtaining and using food cannot be greater than the energy derived from these foods (Odum 1971). These constraints underlie the concept of net energy (Odum 1971) and input–output or cost–yield models (Lee 1969) which may be applied to the subsistence of all organisms. Combined, these concepts form the fundamental principle used to define the geographic limits of a catchment area (Higgs and Vita-Finzi 1972). The basic assumption in defining a human catchment area is that a round trip of over about 10 km to obtain food and return with it to the occupation site is too costly in terms of energy expenditure. The catchment area is usually called home range when it is applied to other animals.

"The aim of the site catchment analysis when applied to a prehistoric site is to assess the resource potential of the area exploited from that site [Higgs 1975:223]." That resource potential is not static and requires a harmony between the optimum time to harvest each resource and the readiness of the people to exploit a changing series of resources. This harmony can be achieved by scheduling (Flannery 1968). This presupposes a changing array of usable resources and decisions on which to exploit. These scheduling decisions are based on a body of knowledge of the environment and reconnaissance information about the current state of each resource.

Knowledge of the environment represents information accumulated over the years, about where plants and animals can be found and at what time of day and times during the year they are most easily obtained. The early development of calendrical notations aided memory by charting the passage of time from the availability of one resource to another.

The survival and well being of the society often depends on scheduling decisions. An apparent lack of a strategy, based on knowledge of where game is located, is a mechanism by which hunting is randomized (Moore 1969). Divination is one such mechanism. By allowing pure chance, the pattern of cracks in a burned scapula for instance, to dictate the area in which to seek game, the hunter ensures that one game population will not become overexploited or excessively wary due to repeated hunting. This means of deciding where to seek game is probably rarely practiced (Vollweiler 1978). Most procurement strategies are based on an intimate knowledge of the location and availability of food resources, and such knowledge is acted upon. Knowledge, such as the probability that King salmon will ascend the Klamath River in the winter (December to February), that hickory nuts (*Carya glabra*) will ripen in the fall (September to October), and that corn will produce a crop in 90 days from the time it is planted, is used in developing procurement strategies.

Models of optimization have been proposed in studies of food selection. These optimization models differ in defining which aspects of the procurement strategy are maximized and which are minimized. Optimization may be viewed in economic terms where costs are minimized and income maximized. In nutritional terms, the calories would be maximized and work, or calories expended, would be minimized. Viewed from another perspective, the strategy may be to satisfy caloric needs while minimizing the work, measured in caloric or time expenditure, needed to achieve caloric sufficiency. Finally, other factors may be introduced into the optimization strategy; for example, not only work but also risk may be minimized and calories of particular food species may be favored for reasons other than purely dietary ones. Thus, models of optimization are complex and differ according to what factors are minimized and maximized. In any one procurement system, subsistence strategies may shift from one model of optimization to another.

The economic strategies have been analyzed in view of their optimizing efficiency. A game theoretical approach has been used in an analysis of decision making by Jamaican fisherman who pit their success in trapping fish against the unpredictably destructive forces of the sea (Davenport 1960). Along the Jamaican coast, fish caught outside the reef are generally more valuable; however, this advantage must be balanced against the greater danger to the fisherman and his equipment encountered while fishing outside the reef. Some fishermen set their traps exclusively inside the reef for a lower yield than would be obtained outside the reef, but this is compensated by exposure to less danger from unpredictable ocean currents. Other fishermen combine fishing strategies to trapping both inside and outside the reef. The game theoretical prediction for the optimum combination of fishing strategies is very close to the observed pattern of fishing. Apparently, the Jamaican fishermen empirically discovered a winning strategy against the "moves" of the opponent, which in this case is the sea.

A similar approach has been used to test the choices made by farmers from the western Ghanaian village of Jantilla in the combination of crops to plant to ensure a sufficient harvest despite unpredictable drought. They have five staple crops that have different resistance to drought and can be planted in various combinations to ensure survival under any environmental conditions. In another example, the choices faced by southern Ghanaian cattle traders in marketing their livestock also lend themselves to a game theoretical or linear analysis. These cattle traders drive their stock to distant markets in the hopes that the higher prices at these markets will offset the risk of cattle losses that may result from being driven long distances through drought-stricken areas (Gould 1969).

The hypothesis that a prehistoric foodway, as reflected by the plant and animal remains, will show a maximization of caloric capture for minimum caloric expenditure requires a number of assumptions. An estimation must be made of the amount of calories potentially provided by the plant and animal used. The calories expended in different subsistence activities must also be estimated. These estimates must then be correlated with the size of the population and the length of their occupation represented by the archeological deposit. With these estimates and their range of error, a strategy of work optimization can be theorized.

A theoretical model of the optimal combination of foods, in terms of minimizing energy required to obtain them and maximizing calories and essential nutrients, may be determined by linear programming. Such a program will take into account the resource availability and its energetic cost and nutrient requirements of the human population. Validation of the theoretically ideal combination can then be made by a comparison with the combination of resources reconstructed from archeological remains. Such a comparison was made between the theoretical model of optimum combination of food resources that could be obtained in the middle Ohio Valley and the reconstructed combination of foods used by the late Woodland and early Fort Ancient people of the Leonard Haag site (Reidhead and Limp 1974). The theoretical model of optimization and the reconstructed use of foods by these prehistoric people differed in some respects. These people did not use mussels and fish as much as the optimization model predicted, but they used nuts more than was predicted. Otherwise the choices of resources used and the priorities by which they were ranked by the prehistoric people is very close to that predicted by modern analysts.

In view of the observed deviations, was an optimal strategy used in the procurement pattern of the prehistoric people inhabiting the Leonard Haag site? A distinction must be made in the perceived goals of the optimization strategy. A commercial strategy usually attempts to achieve the greatest possible returns for the cost input. The objective of the Jamaican fishermen is to get as large and as valuable a catch as is possible with the means at their disposal. Another objective of an optimization strategy is to gear the returns to, in this case, the amounts and kinds of food required to provide the caloric and nutrient needs of the population. This minimization of work for sufficient calories and nutrients has been called the Simon satisficer criterion of the decision-making process (Jochim 1976). Other needs and desires may modify strict adherence to an optimization strategy. Animals provide fur, hide, feathers, bone, and teeth, as well as meat and fat. These products, rather than being strictly nutritional sources, may have an overriding influence on the choices made in the procurement pattern. Some of the differences seen between the reconstructed Leonard Haag site subsistence and the predictive model derived from linear programming may be accounted for by the value placed on some of the resources chosen other than their nutritive contribution.

In a real world situation, it is likely that a combination of these strategies may be used. A subsistence farmer may work to maximize his crops' harvest while hunting only sufficient game to provide a protein supplement to the diet. Such a strategy is described as "garden hunting" inferred from the Cerro Brujo site on the Caribbean coast of Panama (Linares 1976). Similar to many current inland South American groups, such as the Guaymi and Cuna Indians of Panama, the prehistoric inhabitants of Cerro Brujo were primarily agriculturalists. Hunting was basically a by-product of gardening. The cultivated fields and patches of second growth attracted deer, agouti, and collared peccary, which were hunted for the protection of the crops. Clearly subsistence systems are not simple but involve changing priorities to adjust to a dynamic world.

Scheduling and the strategy of optimization are also central to a procurement system of people who are nomadic, migratory, or transhumant. People who are not sedentary must schedule their movements to ever new sets of resources. Such movements of populations or parts of populations are often associated with the migratory patterns of herd animals. Human activity may be designed either to intercept the migratory routes of animals such as caribou or to move domestic herd animals such as llamas to more favorable pastures. Moves are also made to take advantage of the resources in a different habitat or life zone. For this reason, there is archeological evidence and ethnographic substantiation for seasonal occupation of coastal locations.

Archeological evidence for the periodic occupation of a site is usually based on seasonal indicators. Indicators that provide clues to seasonal use of animals and plants are fruits, nuts, seeds, the remains of newborn animals whose reproductive season is known, or the remains of migratory animals, such as migratory birds. The recovery of such seasonal remains do not necessarily mean that the site was unoccupied during the rest of the year. An accumulation of evidence all pointing to use of a number of resources during a single season may, however, be suggestive of seasonal occupation of the site.

Another way the constraints of the environment may be outwitted is by storage of seasonally available foods. Dried grains and nuts are easily stored. Domestic or tamed animals may also be viewed as storages of readily available food. Such storage can provide a cushion against the lean times of the year, providing stability in the food quest. Some types of small scale or short term storage have been in existence a long time, although food storage is usually associated with complex societies where such storage is important in supplying food to concentrations of people.

SUPPLYING FOOD TO CONCENTRATIONS OF PEOPLE

The nutritional requirements of dense concentrations of people usually exceed the carrying capacity of locally available resources. An exception to this is observed when the site is located near a very productive habitat, such as those that are found along the northwest coast of the United States or the coast of Peru. Concentrations of fishes, aquatic mammals, and shore birds, fed by the upwelling of nutrient rich waters, exist in these areas. In those places where the nutrients flow to the human occupants, the carrying capacity is very high. The concentration of food resources available along the coast of Peru has been proposed as a contributing factor to the development of the complex civilization in the Andes (Moseley 1975).

Spatial spread of communities can be seen as an adaptation to the fact that the productivity of most areas is not equally high. Food resources is one of the factors influencing settlement patterns. Settlement patterns and isolation of the factors determining these patterns have come under intensive study. In studies of the Mesoamerican village (Flannery 1976), at least two types of settlement patterns are observed: the linear growth of settlements along a river and its tributaries, and a dispersed pattern with a regularity in the distances between sites of different size and function.

The influence of food resources has been proposed as a determining factor in the maintenance of a buffer or contested zone between some tribal territories. The land between traditional territories occupied by the Sioux and the Chippewa tribes was contested and thus uninhabited between 1780 and 1850 (Hickerson 1965). During that time, this zone of prime deer habitat served as a reservoir for this most important game animal. A comparable buffer zone exists between wolf-pack territories (Mech 1979). The infrequent use of these buffer zones by wolves fosters the survival of deer inhabiting these zones and is reflected in the greater longevity of deer living in these zones. Thus, here again we can see an example of the effect of food resources upon settlement pattern.

The maintenance of dense concentrations of people under most circumstances requires extra human effort. Either the productivity of the land adjacent to the occupation site must be increased, or the territory available to support the community must be expanded. Agriculture is a means of increasing the productivity of edible and acceptable food. Trade, tribute, and taxes are ways in which the support area can be enlarged.

Net food yields (kcal/m²/year) of a given piece of land vary greatly. Productivity is influenced by a combination of soil fertility, rainfall regimes, and the agricultural practices. A comparison of the net food yields derived from gathering and different types of agriculture shows a manifold increase in food yields under different agricultural systems (Figure 8.1). The reduction of limiting factors of the environment by irrigation of dry land, drainage of flooded land, increasing soil nutrients by mulching and fertilization increases the energy flow and thereby the subsequent agricultural output. The "green revolution" and agribusiness achieve their highest yields when subsidies are in the forms of improved plant genotypes, fertilizers, pest control, and mechanized irrigation, planting, and harvesting.

Agricultural practices not subsidized by fossil fuels may also differ widely in their net productivity. Boserup (1965) in her stimulating book on *The Conditions of Agricultural Growth* identifies three broad types of agriculture: (*a*) forest or bush clearing with fire, and planting with a digging stick; (*b*) hoe cultivation; and (*c*) plough cultivation, usually involving a draft animal. The intensity of land use varies under these systems. The least intensive use of the land is known as forest–fallow cultivation, where 1 or 2 years of successive cultivation are followed by a period of fallow of at least 20 years. More intensive cultivation decreases the length of the fallow until

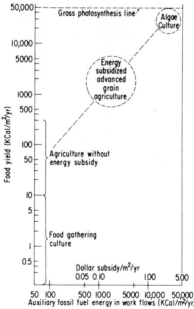

Figure 8-1. Net food yields to man as a function of the subsidy of fossil fuel industries (reprinted by permission of John Wiley and Sons Inc. from *Environment, power, and society* by Howard T. Odum 1971:131).

the most intensive multicropping system in which a plot may be planted with two or three successive crops in 1 year is reached. These are means by which the net productivity of the land may be increased, making it possible to support concentrations of population.

A trade network, market system, and the institution of tribute payment and taxes are the means by which nutrients produced or obtained flow from outlying areas to population centers. Just as with some agricultural systems, such as irrigation, mechanisms of distribution require a degree of control usually associated only with complex social organization. In the one case, control is of the flow and distribution of water to the agricultural fields, and in the other, control ensures the payment of tribute or exchange to the central concentration of the controlling population. An additional benefit of a tribute system to a concentrated population is that it not only expands the territory exploited by a concentration of people, but by doing so assures that a diversity of resources will be provided and a safety measure in times of regional shortages resulting from crop failures, droughts, and other calamities.

BALANCED DIET

Both cultural and physiological mechanisms are called into play in order to ensure balanced nutrition for the individual. Cultural mechanisms for promoting an adequate nutrition involve food preparation and storage, as well as population control. Physiological adaptations are means of reducing the food requirements of the individual and consequently of the population. By a combination of these means, people have adapted to periods of scarcity and to regions which lack important food resources.

One aspect of a procurement system that may affect the nutritional level of the diet is the diversity of plants and animals obtained. The greater this diversity is, the greater the chances are of including in the diet the full range of necessary chemical molecules in ratios suitable for optimum nutrition.

Mass production either by natural systems or by man's industry requires focus and effort on one crop and one kind of yield. Unhappily the change of many systems from diversified natural ones to specialized modern mass production has diminished the relative protein production and has raised the specter of malnutrition. If the carrying capacity of the land increases for carbohydrates and fat without the protein flow also being augmented, a new limiting factor for man develops, one that was not so often as critical in the earlier systems. Species diversity is necessary for nutrition, but with diversity the advantages of mass production are lost. The variety of nature's original habitats provided man with many foods when he was a small part of the system. Later when his agriculture was concentrated on a few plants and replaced nature with a greater net yield of food, his carrying capacity increased but some of the energy converted to increased yield was at the expense of the former diversification. To supply the nutritional diversity again requires an energy expenditure for diversity, either through transportation of products from elsewhere or through local rediversification [From Odum, H.T. *Environment, power, and society,* © 1971 by Wiley, New York, p. 121.]

Diversity in the diet does not necessarily guarantee adequate nutrition. Studies of the dietary diversity and the nutrient intake of the sea-turtle fishing Miskito Indians on the Nicaraguan coast indicate that diversity and optimum nutrition go hand in hand only after caloric requirements are met (Cattle 1976). Once the energy needs are filled, then maximization of the number of food resources tend to increase the likelihood of obtaining the diversity of nutrients required for a balanced diet. Apparently, the subsistence system of the Miskito Indians has been disrupted by the exploitation of a key resource, the sea turtles, by the commercial interests of the developed nations. The economic system of Miskito Indians has been thrown into disequalibrium, and, therefore, the diversity in their diet reflects "food scrounging" rather than an efficient exploitation. This sort of effect, scrounging for food, might be expected in situations when the adaptive subsistence pattern was disrupted by such forces as acculturation, internal social breakdown, or environmental calamity.

Diversity in the procurement system usually has a beneficial effect on the nutritive quality of the diet. Food storage and preparation are also commonly used to enhance the nutritive qualities of the diet by spreading the benefits of a seasonal food over a larger part of the year. The great variety of different methods of preparing food are aimed at making their nutrients more readily available. Grating, grinding, and milling foods mechanically breaks them up into finer particles that can be processed further or can be more easily chewed if it is eaten directly. The advantage of eating foods that are reduced to finer particles is that the protective husk of grains is removed and more surface is exposed so that digestion, the action of salivary amylase, may begin directly in the mouth. Some processing techniques involve leaching tannin out of acorn meal, expressing hydrocyanic acid from grated manioc, and cooking or fermenting ground corn. By doing so, these staples are not only made more palatable, but are also converted to a more digestible form, or even detoxified, making available an excellent carbohydrate source from an otherwise toxic plant, such as manioc. The traditional processing of maize with alkali, which is adhered to by so many people who consume large amounts of maize, is shown to improve the amino-acid balance of the maize. By such treatment, the dangers of the deficiency disease, pellagra, are avoided. When the alkali-treated maize is combined in its traditional pattern with beans, squash, chilis, and meat, the optimum combination of nutrients is achieved. These are but a few examples of ways in which the nutritive qualities of food are enhanced.

Other ways of ensuring adequate nutrition for the survival of a social group are directed toward the control of the numbers of mouths to be fed. Population pressure is a prime cause of disequilibrium in an adapted subsistence system. The response of a population whose nutrient requirements exceed the carrying capacity of its territory, due either to population growth or to resource failure, will be an attempt to recreate an equilibrium by either increasing the available resources, or decreasing the nutrient requirements through population control. Various forms of population control have their own costs, which each population will attempt to minimize, while retaining for itself the greatest degree of biological flexibility.

Five levels of population control can be identified: (a) social and territorial behavior; (b) reproductive behavior; (c) gestation and term; (d) growth and socialization; and (e) longevity and mortality. At the first level of social and territorial behavior, disequilibrium with the environment is corrected by alteration of the population's size and structure to reduce the nutrient requirements. The most common example of this is migration, complete or partial, from the group's own territory to one of more abundant resources. Other behavioral strategies within this category are alterations in courtship practices, incest taboos, and marriage regulations which will suppress matings and marriage, and consequently fertility. These strategies are the least costly to the population since no lives are lost, and are the most flexible since population size is least affected and can quickly be remobilized for reproduction when adequate nutrients are supplied.

At the level of reproductive behavior, the strategy is to modify the risk of exposure to conception, thereby reducing fertility. This can be done by imposing sexual taboos, postpartum or others, by prolonged breast feeding, by regulating sexual techniques, and by the use of artificial birth-control devices, commercial or natural. By using a combination of these techniques—prolonged lactation until the child is 3 years of age or older, and intercourse taboos—the birth of a child can be spaced to occur only every 4 to 5 years during the child-bearing period (Neel 1970). At this level, cost is still low, since pregnancy has been avoided, not wasted, and flexibility is retained.

Study of the physiological cycles of the Kalahari San has demonstrated that those living by hunting and gathering show a clear pattern of seasonal births (Wilmsen 1978). Not only are births concentrated in one season, but this season corresponds with the season when food is most plentiful. Once these people move into an economy dependent on domestic plants and animals, this annual reproductive cycle ceases. Such seasonality would clearly be an advantage in reducing the risk of pregnancy.

The strategy of population control through manipulation of gestation and term involves lowering the probability of successful pregnancy and live birth. Abortion and infanticide are the most highly visible of these techniques. Whereas an infant or fetus whose requirements threaten the society's economic equilibrium may be actively killed, neglect of the pregnant woman, through inadequate diet, and exposure to stress and disease, will have the same effects by increasing the frequency of miscarriage, stillbirth, and infants of low birthweight and birth defects who will not survive. Infanticide, when it is practiced, is often directed toward female children, deformed children, one of a pair of twins, or children born in too close succession to an older sibling (Neel 1970). This level of population control is more costly to the population, since the nutrients invested in the fetus in the early months of life are lost with its death. Nevertheless, flexibility is retained, since within months, the female can become pregnant again.

The control of growth and socialization permits population control through the manipulation of the degree and spread of physical and behavioral maturity. The lack of availability of resources will reduce the speed of physical growth, resulting in short-for-age and thin-for-height children who also have poor resistance to disease. Their mortality rate from common childhood diseases will be higher than for well-nourished children, and benign neglect of the sickly child will permit its death, while support efforts are concentrated on the other members of the family. These techniques are costly since many calories have been invested in the children before their death. Survivors of severe malnutrition may be permanently stunted, reducing their work efficiency, and in the case of females, reducing their future performance as mothers. Furthermore, flexibility is lowered for the population, since replacement of children will take years to accomplish.

The manipulation of longevity and mortality to achieve population control is the most costly to a population. Mortality can be increased and longevity decreased through starvation, either active or passive, through exposure to disease, and through warfare, homicide, suicide, and senilicide. Obvious costly in terms of previous caloric investments, longevity and mortality manipulation also reduces a population's flexibility, since adults of reproductive age are lost, reducing both its capacity to reproduce itself, and to produce food for its remaining members.

These are but a few means by which societies have adapted culturally to ensuring adequate diets for the survival of the cultural group. A number of physiological adaptations have permitted survival during feast and famine conditions or in areas where certain nutrients are in chronically short supply. As we have seen, a way of avoiding famine during periods of food scarcity is by storing food. These storages are usually thought of as containers of grain, jars of oil, dried, salted or smoked fish and meat, or livestock in corrals. Another way of storing nutrient is by accumulations of fat on the body, often the buttocks, during times when food is plentiful. These fat accumulations can be drawn upon during times of food scarcity. Such times of food scarcity may occur on a regular seasonal cycle, during periodic breakdown in procurement, and during population dispersal. Relative food scarcity may also be the result of temporary high-population nutrient requirements, such as during brush clearing or harvesting, or high individual requirements, such as pregnancy. The tendency of, for example Polynesians, to store body fat may result from the selection for those who could survive the long ocean voyages that were taken in the populating of the Polynesian Islands (Diamond 1977). Such an adaptation may be akin to the storage of fat by migrating birds or hibernating bears.

The human body can also store other nutrients in a similar fashion. The human muscles are deposits of protein in somewhat the same way that fat represents stores of energy. During times of need, the protein stored in the muscles can be broken down for either energy, or for amino acids, the particular catabolic pathway dependent on the metabolic requirement.

The bones represent calcium stores which can be drawn upon in the face of dietary scarcity or during high calcium requirements, such as pregnancy or lactation. The fat-soluble vitamins and iron can also be stored, to be retrieved when needed. The human body can also respond to irregular shortages and excesses of most nutrients. By excreting excessive intakes of nutrients, and reducing the losses of nutrients in short supply, the body can maintain homeostasis despite fluctuating intakes. In the case of some nutrients, the body also will absorb more readily those of which the body has need, further facilitating the maintenance of nutrient balance. Reduction of caloric losses during shortages can be achieved by the reduction of activity levels. The rate of growth in children may also be reduced in order to minimize caloric requirements.

An adaptation to persistent nutritional stress, particularly inadequate amounts of protein is a reduction in body size.

> The proportional reduction in body size in all members of a population where protein resources are severely restricted would be adaptive in the sense that more individuals could survive on the available resources, each individual possessing a proportionately small amount of metabolizing tissue with a concomitant reduction in nutritional requirement [Stini 1971:1027]."

This is seen more often as an example of plasticity of the human body rather than a genetic adaptation (Stini 1971).

An example of this may be seen in the skeletal data of prehistoric populations. The projected stature, based on skeletal measurements of prehistoric Mexican and Guatemalan populations, indicates populations of reduced height. The greatest reduction in size comes at a time, the Classic Period, and at a place, central and southern Mesoamerica, that correlates with dependence on intensive food production for subsistence. The hypothesis that inadequate nutrition accompanied the shift from a hunting and a gathering subsistence pattern to an intensive agricultural way of life is further supported by dental and bone abnormalities associated with malnutrition (Nickens 1976). These abnormalities (osteoporotic pitting, porotic hyperostosis, a peridontal degeneration, caries, enamel hypoplasia, etc.) point to a diet deficient in protein, vitamins, and minerals, and high in carbohydrates. If the argument that decrease in stature is an adaptive response to an inadequate diet holds true, then reduction in body size and, therefore, food requirements can only go part of the way to stave off the ravages of severely imbalanced nutrition.

Adaptations to chronic shortages of particular dietary constituents have made it possible for human beings to survive in marginal areas under conditions of nutritional stress. In the Arctic, carbohydrates, the primary precursors of glucose, are scarce. Eskimos live in this region and depend almost exclusively (over 90% of their diet) on meat and fat for food. As a result of selection, Eskimos are genetically adapted to a diet low in carbohydrates by a highly efficient system for glyconeogenesis, which allows the production of glucose from protein and fat (Draper 1977; Lieberman 1976). Another example of stress is that of salt balance. In hot tropical regions, such as parts of Africa, where salt is in short supply, physiological mechanisms for reducing the concentration of sweat and urine sodium, thereby conserving salt, are of adaptive advantage (Gleibermann 1973). Natural selection acting upon renal–adrenal salt-saving mechanisms has conferred an advantage to hunting–gathering peoples of tropical Africa in maintaining their salt balance. These physiological means of avoiding nutritional stress are highly adaptive under the circumstances in which they were selected.

People whose genotype includes adaptation to nutritional stress show imbalances when these stresses are removed. For example, Eskimos adapted to a low carbohydrate diet, by the mechanism of converting protein and fat to glucose, will suffer from obesity when put on a high carbohydrate diet. Likewise, people adapted to conserving salt tend to suffer from hypertension when put on a Western diet with moderate salt. These diseases have been called hyperefficiency diseases, because they result from a "thrift" genotype adapted for survival under nutritional stress.

Diabetes may represent such a hyperefficiency disease (Neel 1962). Diabetes, which results from an insulin deficiency, affects few young people, but rapidly increases in frequency after the age of 50, especially among the obese. Insulin insufficiency prevents sugar from being broken down and absorbed into the cells. Consequently sugar remains in the blood, and may even spill over into the urine if blood sugar levels are high. Diabetes may have evolved as a "thrifty gene" that permitted the conversion of small amounts of excess sugar into fat, but which still retained sugar in the blood to prevent hypoglycemia during what may have been long periods between meals.

With the continuous consumption of a great number of excess calories, especially in the form of carbohydrates and sugars, those individuals carrying the genes for low insulin production find themselves with a hyperefficient trait, which can be harmful, especially without dietary modification.

In conclusion, the satisfaction of nutritional needs are complex, as both physiological and cultural adaptations are involved. The plasticity of these adaptations has made it possible for human beings to cope with the problems and take advantage of the potentials met in all inhabited parts of the world.

Essential for life, food also plays a vital role in cementing human relationships. The most basic human trait of sharing food helps to hold the family unit together. Food and drink are used to seal the bonds between nations. The sharing of food and drink may be highly symbolic, as it is in the Catholic sacrament of communion.

Prehistoric remains can never fully reflect the true extent of the complexity of the prehistoric foodway. However, the role of nutrition is so basic to human existence, it is better to attempt to get a glimpse and accept this view as incomplete rather than to not look at all. Many techniques have been described that are aimed at focusing on this glimpse into the past. Other new and innovative approaches are needed to improve the accuracy of our perceptions.

Appendix:
Legal Considerations Relating to the Collection, Possession, and Transportation of Biological and Archeological Specimens

Complex laws and regulations limit the collection, possession, and transportation of biological specimens, such as skeletons used for comparative purposes, and biological remains from archeological sites, such as human and animal skeletons, shells, and seeds. The complexity is attributable to jurisdictional, substantive, and interpretive variations. Conflicts occur within a given nation between local (county, state, province) and national laws. National attitudes in return may conflict with international legal concepts, compounded by different approaches to preservation in developed and Third World areas. Bilateral and multilateral conventions and treaties have helped resolve some of these conflicts, but they additionally create new conflicts. There also exist substantive differences; definable jurisdictions promote preservation legislation seeking different goals, using different methods to achieve those goals, and following different criteria used to measure success of adopted modes of control. Finally, variations exist in the methodology of interpretation of laws and regulations, partially due to fundamental differences in the several legal traditions which have approached the issue, and partially due to procedural variations. Despite these complexities, it is most important to achieve a level of compliance with both the letter and spirit of these laws designed to protect natural resources. Outlined below is a brief description of the principal laws, to which states or nations are parties, which govern the collection, possession, and transportation of plant and animal specimens and archeological remains as of 1979.

These laws often provide for the adoption of periodic regulations, which may further restrict collection. Interpretive decisions and rulings will also affect the status at a given time. Collectors are consequently advised to familiarize themselves with current laws and regulations, on a local, state, national, and international level before they begin to collect.

Laws pertaining to the collection, possession, and transportation of plant and animal specimens:

1. *Local and state laws.* These laws regulate what, how, and when certain specimens may be collected. Specimens of game animals and fish may further be subject to county and state hunting and fishing regulations. State endangered-species acts protect all of those species identified as endangered by the Federal Endangered Species Act, as well as species locally considered endangered or threatened.

2. *Federal laws.* Federal laws restrict what specimens may be collected and where collecting is limited or prohibited. They also coordinate with local and state laws, to assure compliance with legitimate local interests.

The Federal Endangered Species Act of 1973, which constituted the United States ratification of the 1973 Convention on International Trade in Endangered Species of Wild Fauna and Flora, identifies specific classes of flora and fauna for protection, and constitutes an important international agreement recognizing that effective protection must be accomplished on a global scale.

The United States additionally regulates the collection, preservation, and transportation of plant and animal specimens by separate acts such as the Marine Mammal Protection Act, Migratory Bird Act, Bald Eagle Act, and the prohibition of collection of all plants and animals in wildlife sanctuaries, refuges, critical habitats, and National Parks (Bird Preservation Trespass Act and Environmental Protection Act). The Lacey Act, which regulates commerce, prohibits the movement of any plant, animal, or portion thereof obtained in violation of any local, state, or foreign wildlife regulation. In addition to the Lacey Act, there exists a number of import and export regulations applicable to flora and fauna.

Detailed information about these wildlife regulations and the procedures for obtaining permits is available from: Director, U.S. Fish and Wildlife Service, U.S. Department of the Interior, 1717 H. Street, N.W., Washington, D.C. 20240. The central agency in each state that should be contacted for information about state regulations and permits is listed in the Conservation Directory, updated annually and published by the National Wildlife Federation, Washington, D.C.

3. *International laws and bilateral and multilateral conventions and treaties.* Collection, possession and, most importantly, transportation of biological and archeological specimens may have international aspects that are regulated by a number of treaties, conventions, and laws. In addition to the 1973 Convention on International Trade in Endangered Species of Wild Fauna and Flora, the United States participates in such agreements as migratory bird treaties with Canada and Mexico, the Migratory and Endangered Bird Treaty with Japan, the Convention on Nature Protection and Wildlife Preservation in the Western Hemisphere, the International Convention for the High Seas Fisheries of the North Pacific Ocean, and other international agreements.

Detailed information about the documentation required for the importation of endangered species may be obtained from: Chief, Wildlife Permit Office, U.S. Fish and Wildlife Service, U.S. Department of the Interior, 1717 H. Street, N.W., Washington, D.C. 20240.

Laws pertaining to biological materials from archeological sites:

1. *Local and state laws.* Excavation and collection is subject to compliance with real property laws, requiring permission to undertake archeological projects. Where the project is on state land, the proper state authority must grant approval. It is prohibited to excavate human burials from a known cemetery or mortuary.

2. *Federal laws.* National laws, in the United States or a foreign nation, may govern excavations by persons seeking archeological specimens. National laws are particularly restrictive in many Third World nations which are rich in cultural properties, and archeological projects may be limited to participation by citizens of that nation. In the United States federal laws, such as the Antiquity Act and Historic Sites Act, are designed to protect sites that are of significance to cultural heritage and are located on public lands. Excavation permits must be obtained from appropriate governmental authorities in all countries.

3. *International laws.* The 1970 UNESCO Convention on the Means of Prohibiting and Preventing the Illicit Import, Export and Transfer of Ownership of Cultural Property, which has not been the subject of implementing legislation in the United States, is nevertheless the most important international convention regulating the flow of materials from archeological sites. The United States does participate in several bilateral agreements, such as the 1971 Treaty of Co-operation with the United Mexican States Providing for the Recovery and Return of Stolen Archaeological, Historical and Cultural Properties. Customs officials have the responsibility of identifying and investigating violations of these treaties.

References that outline these regulations in greater detail are as follows:

Burnham, Bonnie
  1974   *The protection of cultural property.* International Council of Museums. Tunisia: Ceres Productions.
Meyer, K.
  1973   *The plundered past.* New York: Atheneum.
Nafziger, J. A. R.
  1976   UNESCO-Centered management of international conflict over cultural property. *Hastings Law Journal 27:*1051.
Poirier, B. W. (director)
  1977   *Archaeological and historical investigations for energy facilities: A state of the art report.* Virginia: Iroquois Research Institute.
Rogers, W.
  1973   The legal response to the illicit movement of cultural property. *Law & Policy in International Business 5:*923.

References

Alfin-Slater, R. B. and H. J. Deuel, Jr.
  1960 The absorption, digestion and metabolism of fats and of related lipids. In *Modern nutrition in health and disease,* 2nd ed., edited by M. G. Wohl and R. S. Goodhart. Philadelphia: Lea & Febiger. Pp. 172–216.

Angress, S., and C. A. Reed
  1962 An annotated bibliography on the origin and descent of domestic mammals. 1900–1955. *Fieldiana: Anthropology* 54(1):5–143.

Antonini, G. A., K. C. Ewel, and H. M. Tupper
  1975 *Population and energy: A systems analysis of resource utilization in the Dominican Republic.* Latin American Monograph (2nd series) no. 14. Gainesville: Univ. Presses of Florida.

Armitage, P. L.
  1975 The extraction and identification of opal phytoliths from teeth of ungulates. *Journal of Archaeological Science* 2(3):187–197.

Asch, N. B., R. I. Ford, and D. L. Asch
  1972 Paleoethnobotany of the Koster Site. *Illinois State Museum Report of Investigation* 6(24):1–34.

Auffenberg, W.
  1963 The fossil snakes of Florida. *Tulane studies in Zoology* 10(3):131–216.

Bailey, G. N.
  1975 The role of molluscs in coastal economics: The result of midden analysis in Australia. *Journal of Archaeological Science* 2(1):45–62.

Beck, C. W.
  1974 Archeological chemistry. *Advances in Chemistry Series* No. 138. American Chemical Society of Washington, D.C.

179

Binford, L. R., and J. B. Bertram
  1977   Bone frequencies—and attritional processes. In *For theory building in archaeology: Essays on faunal remains, aquatic resources, spatial analysis, and systematic modeling,* edited by L. R. Binford. New York: Academic Press, pp. 77–153.

Blakely, R. L.
  1977   Sociocultural implications of demographic data from Etowah, Georgia. *In Biocultural adaptation in prehistoric America,* edited by R. L. Blakely. Athens, Ga.: University of Georgia Press. Pp. 45–66.

Bodenheimer, F. S.
  1951   *Insects as human food.* The Hague: W. Junk.

Bogan, A. R., and N. D. Robison
  1978   A history and selected bibliography of zooarchaeology in eastern North America. *Tennessee Anthropological Association* Misc. Paper No. 2.

Bohrer, V. L. and K. R. Adams
  1977   Ethnobotanical techniques and approaches at Salmon Ruin, New Mexico. San Juan Valley Archaeological Project Tech. Series No. 2. *Eastern New Mexico University Contribution in Anthropology 8*(1):1–215.

Boserup, E.
  1965   *The conditions of agricultural growth.* Chicago: Aldine.

Brandt, K.
  1943   Consumption of fats and oils. In *Nutrition and food supply: The war and after,* edited by J. D. Black. *Annals of the American Academy of Political and Social Science, Philadelphia: 225*:210–220.

Brothwell, D., and E. Higgs
  1963   *Science and archaeology: A comprehensive survey of progress and research.* New York: Basic Books.

Brown, A. B.
  1973   *Bone strontium as a dietary indicator in human skeletal populations,* Ph.D. Dissertation, University of Michigan, Ann Arbor.

  1974   Bone strontium as a dietary indicator in human skeletal populations. *Contribution to Geology 13:47–48.*

Brown, A. B., and H. Keyzer
  1978   Sample preparation for strontium analysis of ancient skeletal remains. *Contribution to Geology 16:85–87.*

Brown, A. T.
  1976   The role of dietary carbohydrates in plaque formation and oral disease. In *Present knowledge in nutrition,* 4th ed. New York: The Nutrition Foundation. Pp. 488–503.

Bryant, F. J., and J. F. Loutit
  1961   Human bone metabolism deduced from strontium assays. United Kingdom Atomic Energy Authority Research group Report R-3718, London: H.M. Stationery Office.

Bryant, V. M. Jr.
  1974a   The role of coprolite analysis in archeology. *Bulletin Texas Archaeological Society 45:1–28.*

  1974b   Pollen analysis of prehistoric human feces from Mammoth Cave. In *Archeology of the Mammoth Cave area,* edited by P. J. Watson. New York: Academic Press.

Buikstra, J. E.
  1977   Biocultural dimensions of archeological study: a regional perspective. In *Biocultural adaptation in prehistoric America,* edited by R. L. Blakely. Athens, Ga.: University of Georgia Press. Pp. 67–84.

Burchard, R.
1975   Coca chewing: A new perspective. In *Cannabis and culture*, edited by V. Rubin. The Hague: Mouton.
Burleigh, R., and D. Brothwell
1978   Studies on Amerindian dogs, 1: Carbon isotopes in relation to maize in the diet of domestic dogs from early Peru and Ecuador. *Journal of Archaeological Science* 5:355–362.
Byers, D. S.
1967   *The prehistory of the Tehuacan Valley* (Vol. 1), *Environment and subsistence*. London: Univ. of Texas Press.
Cabrera, A., and J. Yepes
1960   *Maniferos Sud Americanos*. Argentina: Ediar S A Editores.
Caddell, J. L.
1969   Magnesium deficiency in PCM: A follow-up study. *Annals of the New York Academy of Science* 162:874–890.
Callen, E. O.
1963   Diet as revealed by coprolites. In *Science in archeology*, edited by D. Brothwell and E. S. Higgs. London: Thames and Hudson.
1967   Analysis of Tehuacan coprolites. In *The prehistory of the Tehuacan Valley* (Vol. 1). *Environment and subsistence*, edited by D. S. Byers. Austin: Univ. of Texas Press.
Calorie Requirements
1957   F.A.O. Nutritional Study No. 15, p. 10, F.A.O. Rome.
Carlson, D. S., G. J. Armelagos, and D. P. Van Gerven
1974   Factors influencing the etiology of cribra orbitalia in prehistoric Nubia. *Journal of Human Evolution* 3:405–410.
Carter G. F.
1977   The metate: An early grain-grinding implement in the New World. In *Origins of agriculture*, edited by C. A. Reed. The Hague: Mouton Publishers.
Casteel, R. W.
1974   A method for estimation of live weight of fish from the size of skeletal elements. *American Antiquity* 39(1):94–98.
1976a   *Fish remains in archeology and paleo-environmental studies*. London: Academic Press.
1976b   Incremental growth zones in mammals and their archaeological value. *Kroeber Anthropological Society Papers* 547:1–27.
1976–1977 A consideration of the behavior of the Minimum Number of Individuals Index: A problem in faunal characterization. *Ossa* 3/4:141–151.
1977   Characterization of faunal assemblages and the minimum number of individuals determined from paired elements: Continuing problems in archaeology. *Journal of Archaeological Science* 4(2):125–134.
1978   Faunal assemblages and the "Wiegemethode" or weight method. *Journal of Field Archaeology* 5(1):71–77.
Cattle, D. J.
1976   Dietary diversity and nutritional security in a Coastal Miskito Indian Village, Eastern Nicaragua. In *Frontier adaptations in Lower Central America*, edited by M. W. Helms and F. O. Loveland. Philadelphia: ISHI.
Chaplin, R. E.
1971   *The study of animal bones from archaeological sites*. New York: Seminar Press.

Clarke, D. L.
1972 Models and paradigms in contemporary archaeology. In *Models in Archaeology*, edited by D. L. Clarke. London: Menthuen.

Clason, A. T.
1972 Some remarks on the use and presentation of archaeozoological data. *Helinium* 12(2):139–153.
1975 *Archaeozoological Studies*. Papers of the Archaeozoological Conference 1974, held at the Biologisch-Archaeologisch Instituut of the State University of Groningen. Amsterdam: North Holland Publ. Co.

Clason, A. T. and W. Prummel
1977 Collecting, sieving and archaeozoological research. *Journal of Archaeological Science* 4(2):171–175.

Clastres, P.
1972 The Guayaki. In *Hunters and gatherers today*, edited by M. G. Bicchieri. New York: Holt.

Cohan, M. N.
1977 *The food crisis in prehistory: Overpopulation and the origins of agriculture*. New Haven: Yale Univ. Press.

Comar, C. L., L. Russell, and R. H. Wasserman
1957 Strontium-calcium movement from soil to man, *Science 126*, 485–492.

Cook, D. C.
1971 *Patterns of nutritional stress in some Illinois Woodland populations*. Master's Thesis, University of Chicago.
1976 Pathologic states and disease process in Illinois woodland populations: An epidemiologic approach. Ph.D. dissertation, University of Chicago.

Cook, G. C.
1978 Did persistence of intestinal lactase into adult life originate on the Arabian Peninsula? *Man 13*(3):418–427.

Cook, S. F.
1946 A reconsideration of shell mounds with respect to population and nutrition. *American Antiquity 12*:50–53.

Cordano, A., J. M. Baertl, and G. G. Graham
1964 Copper deficiency in infancy. *Pediatrics 34*:324–336.

Crain, J. B.
1971 Human paleopathology: A bibliographic list. *Sacramento Anthropological Society Paper 12*, Sacramento, California.

Cumbaa, S. L.
1972 *An intensive harvest economy in North Central Florida*. Master's thesis, University of Florida, Gainesville.
1973 Subsistence strategy at Venedillo, Sinaloa, Mexico. *West Mexican Prehistory* part 7, mimeo, Anthropology Department, State University of New York at Buffalo.

Darwin, C.
1962 *The voyage of the Beagle*, edited by L. Engel. New York: The Natural History Library Anchor Books, Doubleday.

Davenport, W.
1960 Jamaican fishing: A game theory analysis. *Yale University Publications in Anthropology* No. 59:3–11.

DeBoer, W. R.
1975 The archaeological evidence for manioc cultivation: A cautionary note. *American Antiquity 40*(4):419–433.

DeFoliart, G. R.
 1975   Insects as a source of protein. *Bulletin Entomological Society of America 21*:161–163.

Denevan, W. M.
 1970   Aboriginal drained-field cultivation in the Americas. *Science 169*:647–654.

DeNiro, M. J.and S. Epstein
 1978   Carbon isotopic evidence for different feeding patterns in two hyrax species occupying the same habitat. *Science 201*:906–908.

Deuel, H. J.
 1955   The absorption, digestion and metabolism of fats and related lipids. In *Modern nutrition in health and disease*, edited by M. G. Wohl and R. S. Goodhart. Philadelphia: Lee & Febiger.

Diamond, J. M.
 1977   Colonization cycles in man and beast. *World Archaeology 8*(3):249–261.

Dick, J. L.
 1922   *Rickets*, London: J. Heinemann.

Dimbleby, G. W.
 1967   *Plants and archaeology*. London: Humanities Press.

Donnan, C. B.
 1976   *Moche art and iconography*. Los Angeles, California: UCLA Latin-American Center Publication.

Draper, H. H.
 1977   The aboriginal Eskimo diet in modern perspective. *American Anthropologist 79*:309–316.

Dreizen, S., R. M. Snodgrass, H. Webb-Peploe, and T. D. Spies
 1958   Retarding effect on protracted undernutrition on the appearance of postnatal ossification centers in the hand and wrist. *Human Biology 30*:253–264.

Dreizen, S., C. N. Sparks, and R. E. Stone
 1965   Distribution and disposition of anomalous notches in the nonepiphyseal ends of the human metacarpal shafts, *American Journal of Physical Anthropology 23*:181–188.

Duran, Fray Diego
 1967   *Historia de las Indias de Nuevo Espanz y Islas de Tierra Firma* (Edition introduced by J. F. Ramirez). Mexico: Editora Nacional.

Emory, K. P., W. J. Bonk, and Y. H. Sinoto
 1968   Hawaiian Archaeology Fishhooks. *Bernice P. Bishop Museum Special Publication No. 47.*

Evans, J. G.
 1972   *Land snails in archaeology with special reference to the British Isles*. London: Seminar Press.

Faegri, K. and J. Iversen
 1966   *Textbook of pollen analysis*. 2nd edition. Oxford Press.

Flannery, K. V.
 1968   Archeological systems theory and early Mesoamerica. In *Anthropological Archeology in the Americas*, edited by Betty J. Meggers. Anthropological Society of Washington, Washington, D.C. Pp. 67–87.
 1976   *The early Mesoamerican village*. New York: Academic Press.

Frampton, V. L.
 1975   Effects of handling and storage on seeds. In *Nutritional evaluation of food processing*, 2nd ed., edited by R. Harris and E. Karmas. Westport, Conn.: AVI.

Frazer, J. G.
1959 *The New Golden Bough* (abridged edition). New York: Criterion Books.

Frost, H. M.
1964 Mathematical elements of Lamellar bone remodeling. Springfield, Illinois: Charles C. Thomas.

Gade, D. W.
1975 Plants, man and the land in the Vilcanota Valley of Peru. *Biogeographica VI:* The Hague: W. Junk.

Garn, S. M., and R. S. Baby
1969 Bilateral symmetry in finer lines of increased density. *American Journal of Physical Anthropology 31:89–92.*

Garn, S. M., F. N. Silverman, K. P. Hertzog, and C. G. Rohmann
1968 Lines and bands of increased density, *Medical Radiography and Photography 44:58–59.*

Geiger, E.
1955 Digestion, absorption and metabolism of protein. In *Modern nutrition in health and disease,* edited by M. G. Wohl and R. S. Goodhart. Philadelphia: Lee & Febiger.

Genoves, S. C.
1967 Proportionality of long bones and their relationship to stature among mesoamericans. *American Journal of Physical Anthropology 56:67–78.*

Gifford, D. P. and A. K. Behrensmeyer
1977 Observed formation and burial of a recent human occupation site in Kenya. *Quaternary Research 8:245–266.*

Gifford, E. W.
1916 Composition of California shell mounds. *University of California Publications in American Archaeology and Ethnology 12:1–29.*

Gilbert, B. M.
1973 *Mammalian osteo-archaeology: North America.* Columbia, Missouri: Missouri Archaeological Society.

Gilbert, B. M., L. D. Martin, and H. G. Savage
n.d. *Avian osteo-archeology: North America.* Columbia, Missouri: Missouri Archaeological Society.

Gilbert, R. I.
1975 *Trace element analyses of three skeletal Amerindian populations at Dickson Mounds.* Ph.D. Dissertation, University of Massachusetts, Amherst.

Gilliland, M. S.
1975 *The material culture of Key Marco, Florida.* Gainesville: University Presses of Florida.

Gleiberman, L.
1973 Blood pressure and dietary salt in human populations. *Ecology of Food and Nutrition 2:143–156.*

Gordon, C. C. and J. E. Buikstra
1979 *Soil pH, bone preservation, and sampling bias at mortuary sites.* Paper presented at the 44th annual meeting Society for American Archaeology Vancouver, British Columbia.

Gould, P. R.
1969 Man against his environment: A game theoretical framework. In *Environment and Cultural Behavior,* edited by A. P. Vayda. New York: Natural History Press.

Grayson, D. K.
1973 On the methodology of faunal analysis. *American Antiquity 38*(4):432–439.

Greengo, R. E.
1951 Molluscan species in California shell middens. *University of California Archaeological Survey Report 13:1–29.*

Gregory, W. K.
1933 *Fish skulls* (reissued in 1959 by E. Lundberg, Laural, Fla.) Original publication in *Transactions American Philosophical Society 23(2).*

Guilday, J. E., P. W. Parmalee, D. P. Tanner
1962 Aboriginal butchering techniques at the Eschelman Site (36 La 12) Lancaster County, Pennsylvania. *Pennsylvania Archaeologist: Bulletin of the Society of Pennsylvanian Archaeology 32(2):59–83.*

Gunn, C. R.
1972 Seed collecting and identification. In *Seed Biology,* Vol. 3, edited by T. T. Kozlowski. New York: Academic Press.

Haag, W. G.
1948 An osteometric analysis of some aboriginal dogs. *University of Kentucky Report in Anthropology 7(3):107–264.*

Hall, E. R. and K. R. Kelson
1959 *The mammals of North America.* New York: Ronald Press.

Hargrave, L. L.
1970 Mexican macaws: Comparative osteology and survey of remains from the Southwest. *Anthropological Papers University Arizona Press* No. 20 Tucson, Arizona.
1972 Comparative osteology of the chicken and American grouse. *Prescott College Studies in Biology* No. 1.

Harris, R. S.
1975 General discussion on the stability of nutrients. In *Nutritional evaluation of food processing,* 2nd ed., edited by R. Harris and E. Karmas. Westport, Conn.: AVI.

Harvey, E. B., H. E. Kaiser, and L. E. Rosenberg
1968 *An atlas of the domestic turkey (Meleagris gallopavo): Myology and osteology.* United States Atomic Energy Commission.

Hatch, M. D. and C. R. Slack
1970 Photosynthetic CO_2-fixation pathways. *Annual Review of Plant Physiology 21:*141–162.

Haviland, W. A.
1967 Stature at Tikal: Implications for ancient Maya demography and social organization. *American Antiquity 35:*316–325.

Hegsted, D. M.
1955 Calcium and phosphorus. In *Modern nutrition in health and disease,* edited by M. A. Wahl and R. S. Goodhart. Philadelphia: Lee and Febiger.

Heiser, C. B., Jr.
1973 *Seed to civilization.* San Francisco: W. H. Freeman.

Helbaek, H.
1954 Prehistoric food plants and weeds of Denmark: A survey of archaeo-botanical research 1923–1954. *Danmarks Geoligiske Unders* II No. 80:250–61.

Hickerson, H.
1965 The Virginia deer and intertribal buffer zones in the Upper Mississippi Valley. In *Man, culture, and animals,* edited by Leeds and A. P. Vayda. American Association for the Advancement of Science, publication 78, Washington, D.C.

Higgs, E. S.
1972 *Papers in economic prehistory: Studies by members and associates of the British Academy Major Research Project in the early history of agriculture.* Cambridge, GB: University Press.

1975 *Palaeoeconomy: The second volume of papers in economic prehistory.* Cambridge, GB: University Press.

Higgs, E. S. and C. Vita-Finzi
1972 Prehistoric economies: A territorial approach. In *Papers in economic prehistory,* edited by E. S. Higgs. Cambridge, GB: University Press.

Higham, C.
1968 Size trends in prehistoric European domestic fauna and the problem of local domestication. *Acta Zoologica Fennica 120:*1–21.

Hodges, R. M., N. S. MacDonald, R. Nusbaum, R. Stearns, F. Ezmirlian, P. Spain, and C. MacArthur
1950 Strontium content of human bones. *Journal of Biological Chemistry 185:*519–524.

Horwitt, M. K.
1955 The nature, distribution, absorption, and metabolism of thiamine, riboflavin, and niacin. In *Modern nutrition in health and disease,* edited by M. G. Wohl and R. S. Goodhart. Philadelphia: Lee and Febiger.

Issac, G.
1971 The diet of early man. *World Archaeology 2*(3):278–298.

Jaffee, H. L.
1972 *Metabolic, degenerative and inflammatory diseases of bones and joints.* Philadelphia: Lee and Febiger.

Jarman, H. N., A. J. Legge, and J. A. Charles
1972 Retrieval of plant remains from archaeological sites by froth flotation. In *Papers in economic prehistory,* edited by E. S. Higgs. Cambridge, GB: University Press.

Jochim, M. A.
1976 *Hunter–gatherer subsistence and settlement: A predictive model.* New York: Academic Press.

Karmas, E.
1975 Nutritional aspects of food processing methods. In *Nutritional evaluation of food processing,* 2nd ed., edited by R. Harris and E. Karmas. Westport, Conn.: AVI.

Katz, S. H., M. L. Hediger, and L. A. Valleroy
1974 Traditional maize processing techniques in the New World. *Science 184:*765–773.

Keeley, L. H., and M. H. Newcomer
1977 Microwear analysis of experimental flint tools: A test case. *Journal of Archaeological Science 4*(1):29–62.

Kikuchi, W. K.
1976 Prehistoric Hawaiian fish ponds. *Science 193:*295–299.

Krantz, G. S.
1968 A new method of counting mammal bones. *American Journal of Archaeology 72:*286–288.

Kraybill, N.
1977 Pre-agricultural tools for the preparation of foods in the Old World. In *Origins of agriculture,* edited by C. A. Reed. The Hague: Mouton Publishers.

Krochta, J. M. and B. Feinberg
1975 Effects of harvesting and handling on fruits and vegetables. In *Nutritional evaluation of food processing.* 2nd Ed., edited by R. Harris and E. Karmas. Westport, Conn.: AVI.

Kromer, G. W.
1961 Food fat consumption continues stable. In *1960, Fats and Oils Situation.* FOS-207, Agri-Marketing Service, Agricultural Economics Division, USDA, March, 1961.

Krueger, R. H.
1969 Some long-term effects of severe malnutrition in early life. *Lancet 2:*514.

Kulebakina, L. G.
  1975 Strontium-90 in the cystoseiric biocenosis of the Black Sea shelf zone. In *Self-purification, bioproductivity, and protection of reservoirs and currents of water in the Ukraine,* edited by A. V. Topachevskii. Kiev, USSR: Naukova Dumka Publ.

Kulp, J. L., W. R. Eckelmann, and A. R. Schulert
  1957 Strontium-90 in man. *Science 125* (3241):219–225.

Lachance, P. A.
  1975 Effects of food preparation procedures on nutrient retention with emphasis upon food service practices. In *Nutritional evaluation of food processing,* 2nd ed., edited by R. Harris and E. Karmas. Westport, Conn.: AVI.

Lee, M., and S. M. Garn
  1967 Pseudo-epiphyses or notches in the non-epiphyseal end of metacarpal bones in healthy children. *The Anatomical Record 159:*263–272.

Lee, M., S. M. Garn, and C. G. Rohmann
  1968 Relation of metacarpal notching to stature and maturational status of normal children. *Investigative Radiology 3:*96–102.

Lee, R. B.
  1969 !Kung bushman subsistence: An input–output analysis. In *Environment and cultural behavior,* edited by A. P. Vayda. New York: Natural History Press.

Lee, R. B., and I. DeVore
  1968 *Man the hunter.* Chicago: Aldine Publishing Co.

Lerman, J. C. and J. H. Troughton
  1975 Carbon isotope discrimination by photosynthesis: Implications for the bio- and geosciences. In *Proceedings for the Second International Conference on Stable Isotopes,* edited by E. R. Klein and P. D. Klein.

Lewis, O.
  1960 *Tepoztlan, village in Mexico.* New York: Holt.

Lieberman, L. S.
  1976 Diet, natural selection and adaptation in human populations. Paper presented at 75th annual meeting of the American Anthropological Association, Washington, D.C.

Linares, O. F.
  1976 "Garden Hunting" in the American tropics. *Human Ecology 4*(4):331–349.

Lisker, R., B. Gonzales, and M. Daltabuit
  1975 Recessive inheritance of the adult type of intestinal lactase deficiency. *American Journal of Human Genetics 27:*662–664.

Little, K.
  1973 *Bone behaviour.* London: Academic Press.

Lomax, A., and C. M. Arensberg
  1977 A worldwide evolutionary classification of cultures by subsistence systems. *Current Anthropology 18*(4):659–708.

Lowery, G. H., Jr.
  1974 *The mammals of Louisiana and its adjacent waters.* Baton Rouge Louisiana State University Press.

Matheny, R. T.
  1976 Maya lowland hydraulic systems. *Science 193:*639–646.

McHenry, H.
  1968 Transverse line in long bones of prehistoric California Indians. *American Journal of Physical Anthropology 29:*1–17.

McLean, F. C., and M. R. Urist
  1961 *Bone: An introduction to the physiology of skeletal tissue.* Chicago: Univ. of Chicago Press.

Mech, L. D.
1979 Why some deer are safe from wolves. *Natural History* 88(1):70–77.
Meighan, C. E.
1969 Molluscs as food remains in archaeological sites. In *Science and Archaeology,* edited by D. Brothwell and E. Higgs. Revised edition. London: Thames and Hudson.
Meyer de Schauensee, R.
1970 *A guide to the birds of South America.* Wynnewood, Pennsylvania: Livingston Press.
Mickelson, O., and D. D. Makdani
1975 Factors affecting nutrient metabolism. In *Nutritional evaluation of food processing,* (2nd edition), edited by R. S. Harris and E. Karmas. Westport, Conn.: AVI.
Miller, G. S., and R. Kellogg
1955 List of North American recent mammals. *U.S. National Museum Bulletin* 205, Washington, D.C.
Miller, M. E.
1964 *Anatomy of the dog.* Philadelphia: W.B. Saunders Co.
Molnar, S.
1971 Human tooth wear, tooth function and cultural variability. *American Journal of Physical Anthropology* 34:175–189.
1972 Tooth wear and culture: A survey of tooth functions among some prehistoric populations. *Current Anthropology* 13:511–526.
Montgomery, F. H.
1977 *Seeds and fruits of plants of Eastern Canada and Northeastern United States.* Toronto: Univ. of Toronto Press.
Moore, C. V.
1955 Iron and the essential trace elements. In *Modern nutrition in health and disease,* edited by M. A. Wohl and R. S. Goodhart, Philadelphia: Lee and Febiger.
Moore, O. K.
1969 Divination—New perspective. In *Environment and cultural behavior,* edited by A. P. Vayda. New York: Natural History Press.
Moseley, M. E.
1975 *The maritime foundations of Andean civilization.* California: Cummings Publishing Co.
Murdock, G. P.
1967 *Ethnographic Atlas.* Pittsburgh, Pennsylvania: Univ. of Pittsburgh Press.
Murra, J. V.
1973 Rite and crop in the Inca state. In *Peoples and cultures of native South America,* edited by D. R. Gross. New York: The National History Press Doubleday.
Nash, O.
1945 *Many Long Years Ago.* Boston: Little Brown.
Neale, G.
1968 The diagnosis, incidence and significance of dissacharidase deficiency in adults. *Proceedings of the Royal Society of Medicine* 61:1099–1102.
Neel, J. V.
1962 Diabetes mellitus: a "thrift" genotype rendered detrimental by "progress"? *American Journal of Human Genetics* 14:353.
1970 Lessons from a "primitive" people. *Science* 170(3960):815–822.
Nelson, N. C.
1909 Shell mounds of the San Francisco Bay region. *University of California Publications in American Archaeology and Ethnology* 7:303–356.
1910 The Ellis Landing shell mound. *University of California Publications in American Archaeology and Ethnology* 17:357–426.

Nelson, R. K.
   1969   *Hunters of the northern ice.* Chicago: Univ. of Chicago Press.
Nickens, P. R.
   1976   Stature reduction as an adaptive response to food production in Mesoamerica. *Journal of Archaeological Science 3*:31–41.
Nietschmann, B.
   1973   *Between land and water: The subsistence ecology of the Miskito Indians, Eastern Nicaragua.* New York: Seminar Press.
Noe-Nygaard, N.
   1975   Bone injuries caused by human weapons. In *Archaeozoological Studies,* edited by A. T. Clason. Amsterdam: North Holland Publishing Co.
Odum, H. T.
   1971   *Environment, power, and society.* New York: Wiley.
Odum, J. T.
   1957   Strontium in natural waters. *Texas University Institute of Marine Science Publication, 4*:22–37.
Olsen, S. J.
   1964   Mammal remains from archaeological sites. Part 1 Southwestern and Southeastern United States. *Papers of the Peabody Museum of Archaeology and Ethnology,* Harvard University, Cambridge 56(1).
Ophel, I. L.
   1963   The fate of radiostrontium in a freshwater community. In *Radioecology,* edited by V. Schultz and A. W. Klement. London: Chapman and Hall.
Park, E. A.
   1954   Bone growth in health and disease. *Archives of Diseases in Children 29*:269–281.
   1964   Imprinting of nutritional disturbances on the growing bone. *Pediatrics 33*:915–862.
Park, E. A. and C. P. Richter
   1953   Transverse lines in bone: The mechanism of their development. *Bulletin of Johns Hopkins Hospital 41*:364–388.
Parker, R., and H. Toots
   1970   Minor elements in fossil bone. *Geological Society of America Bulletin 81.*
Parmalee, P. W., and W. E. Klippel
   1974   Freshwater mussels as a prehistoric food resource. *American Antiquity 39*(3):421–434.
Passmore, R., and J. Durnin
   1955   Human energy expenditure. *Physiological Review 35*:801.
Payne, S.
   1972   Partial recovery and sample bias: The results of some sieving experiments. In *Papers in economic prehistory,* edited by E. S. Higgs. Cambridge, GB: University Press.
Pearsall, D. M.
   1978   Phytolith analysis of archeological soils: Evidence for maize cultivation in formative Ecuador. *Science 199*:177–178.
Pedley, T. J.
   1977   *Scale effects in animal locomotion.* London: Academic Press.
Perkins, D. Jr.
   1973   A critique on the methods of quantifying faunal remains from archaeological sites. In *Domesticationsforschung und geschichte der Haustiere,* edited by J. Matolosi. Budapest: Adademiai Kiado.
Perkins, D. Jr., and P. Daly
   1968   A hunter's village in neolithic Turkey. *Scientific American 219*(5):96–106.

Perzigian, A. J.
  1977 Teeth as tools for prehistoric studies. In *Biocultural adaptation in prehistoric America*, edited by R. L. Blakely, Athens, Ga.: University of Georgia Press.
Peterson, R. T.
  1947 *A field guide to the birds*. Boston: Houghton Mifflin.
Pike, R. L., and M. L. Brown
  1967 *Nutrition: An integrated approach*. New York: John Wiley.
Prange, H. D., J. F. Anderson, and H. Rahn
  1979 Scaling of skeletal mass to body mass in birds and mammals. *American Naturalist* 113(1):103–122.
Price, R.
  1966 Fishing rites and recipes in a Martiniquan village. *Caribbean Studies* VI(1):3–24.
Randall, J. E.
  1968 *Caribbean reef fishes*. New Jersey: TFH Publ.
Recommended Dietary Allowances
  1968 Seventh Edition, p. 7. National Academy of Sciences, Washington, D.C.
Reed, C. A.
  1963 Osteo-archaeology. In *Science in Archaeology*. edited by D. Brothwell and E. Higgs. New York: Basic Books.
Reichel-Dolmatoff, G.
  1971 *Amazonian cosmos: The sexual and religious symbolism of the Tukano Indians*. Chicago: Univ. of Chicago Press.
Reidhead, V. A., and W. F. Limp
  1974 Nutritional maximization: A multifaceted nutritional model for archaeological research. Paper presented at 73rd annual meeting of the American Anthropological Association, Mexico City.
Reitz, E. J.
  1979 *Spanish and British subsistence strategies at St. Augustine, Florida, and Frederica, Georgia, between 1563 and 1783*. Ph.D. Dissertation, University of Florida, Gainesville.
Renfrew, J. M.
  1973 *Paleoethnobotany: The prehistoric food plants of the Near East and Europe*. New York: Columbia Univ. Press.
Renfrew, J. M., M. Monk, and P. Murphy
  1975 First aid for seeds. *RESCUE Publication* No. 6, p. 35.
Reynolds, W. W., and W. J. Karlotski
  1977 The allometric relationships of skeleton weight to body weight in teleost fishes: A preliminary comparison with birds and mammals. *Copeia* 1977 (1):160–163.
Rice, E. E.
  1975 Effects of postmortem handling. In *Nutritional evaluation of food processing*, 2nd ed., edited by R. Harris and E. Karmas. Westport, Conn.: AVI.
Rick, A. M.
  1975 Bird medullary bone: A seasonal dating technique for faunal analysts. *Canadian Archaeological Association Bulletin* No. 7, pp. 183–190.
Ricklefs, R. E.
  1973 *Ecology*. Newton, Massachusetts: Chiron Press.
Robson, J. R. K.
  1972 *Malnutrition: Its causation and control*. New York: Gordon and Breach.
Romer, A. S.
  1945 *Vertebrate paleontology*. Chicago: Univ. of Chicago Press.

Rosenthal, H. L.
  1963   Uptake, turnover and transfer of bone seeking elements in fishes. *Annals New York Academy of Science 109:* 278–293.
Roth, W. E.
  1916–1917 An introductory study of the arts, crafts and customs of the Guiana Indians. (1970 reprint.) *U.S. Bureau of American Ethnology* 38th Annual Report.
Rovner, I.
  1971   Potential of opal phytoliths for use in paleoecological reconstruction. *Quaternary Research 1:343–359.*
Ruddle, K.
  1973   The human use of insects: Examples from the Yukpa. *Biotropica 5:94–101.*
Sadek-Kooros, H.
  1972   Primitive bone fracturing: A method of research. *American Antiquity 37:369–382.*
  1975   International fracturing of bone: Description of criteria. In *Archaeozoological Studies,* edited by A. T. Clason. Amsterdam: North-Holland Publ. Co.
Sauer, C. O.
  1952   *Agricultural origins and dispersals.* New York: American Geographic Society.
Schmid, E.
  1972   *Atlas of animal bones for prehistorians, archaeologists and Quaternary geologists.* Amsterdam: Elsevier.
Schoeninger, M. J.
  1979   Dietary reconstruction at Chalcatzingo, a Formative Period site in Morelos, Mexico. *Museum of Anthropology, The University of Michigan,* Technical Reports #9.
Schroeder, H. A., I. H. Tipton, and A. P. Nason
  1972   Trace metals in man: Strontium and barium. *Journal of Chronic Disease 25:491–517.*
Schwager, P. M.
  1968   The frequency of appearance of transverse lines in the tibia in relation to childhood illnesses. Abstracted in *American Journal of Physical Anthropology 29:130.*
Schwarz, H. F.
  1948   Stingless bees (Meliponidae) of the Western Hemisphere. *Bulletin American Museum Natural History 90.*
Scrimshaw, N.
  1966   Effects of the interaction of nutrition and infection in the preschool child. In *Malnutrition in the preschool child,* NAS–NRC, Washington, D.C.
Sebrell, W. H. Jr. and J. J. Haggerty
  1967   *Food and nutrition.* New York: Time–Life Books.
Semenov, S. A.
  1957   *Prehistoric technology.* London: Cory, Adams and Mackay.
Severinghaus, C. W.
  1949   Tooth development and wear as criteria of age in white-tailed deer. *Journal of Wildlife Management 13*(2):195–216.
Shackleton, N. J.
  1973   Oxygen isotope analysis as a means of determining season of occupation of prehistoric midden sites. *Archaeometry, 15:133–141.*
Shawcross, W.
  1967   An investigation of prehistoric diet and economy on a coastal site at Galatea Bay, New Zealand. *Proceedings Prehistoric Society 33:107–131.*
  1972   Energy and ecology: Thermodynamics models in archaeology. In *Models in Archaeology,* edited by D. L. Clarke. London: Methuen.

Shotwell, J. A.

1955 An approach to the paleoecology of mammals. *Ecology* 36:327–337.

1958 Inter-community relationships in Hemphillian (Mid-Pliocene) mammals. *Ecology* 39:271–282.

Simoons, F. J.

1967 *Eat not this flesh: Food avoidance in the Old World.* Madison: Univ. of Wisconsin Press.

Slobodkin, L. B.

1977 Evolution is no help. *World Archaeology* 8(3):332–343.

Smith, B. D.

1975 Middle Mississippi exploitation of animal populations. *Anthropological Papers* No. 57, University of Michigan.

1976 "Twitching": A minor ailment affecting human paleoecological research. In *Cultural change and continuity,* edited by C. E. Cleland. New York: Academic Press.

Smith, C. E.

1971 Preparing herbarium specimens of vascular plants. *Agriculture Information Bulletin* No. 348. Agriculture Research Service USDA.

Somogyi, J. C.

1966 *Antivitamins, bibliothecanutrio et dieta,* Basel: S. Karger.

Soskin, S., and R. Levine

1955 The role of carbohydrates in the diet. In *Modern Nutrition in Health and Disease,* edited by M. G. Wohl and R. S. Goodhart. Philadelphia: Lee and Febiger.

Sowden, E. M., and S. R. Stitch

1957 Trace elements in human tissues, 2. Estimation of the concentration of stable strontium and barium in human bone. *Biochemical Journal,* 67:104–109.

Spier, R. F. G.

1970 *From the hand of man: Primitive and preindustrial technologies.* Boston: Houghton Mifflin.

Steward, J. H.

1974 The Great Basin Shoshonean Indians. An example of a family level of sociocultural integration. In *Man in Adaptation: The cultural present,* edited by Y. A. Cohan. Chicago: Aldine.

Stewart, H.

1977 *Indian fishing: Early methods on the Northwest Coast.* Seattle: Univ. of Washington Press.

Stini, W. A.

1971 Evolutionary implications of changing nutritional patterns in human populations. *American Anthropologist* 73:1019–1030.

Strong, F. M.

1976 Toxicants occurring naturally in foods. In *Present knowledge in nutrition,* 4th ed. New York: The Nutrition Foundation.

Struever, S.

1968 Flotation techniques for the recovery of small-scale archeological remains. *American Antiquity* 33(3):353–362.

Szpunar, C.

1977 *Atomic absorption analysis of archaeological remains: Human ribs from Woodland mortuary sites.* Ph.D. Dissertation, Northwestern University, Evanston, Illinois.

Szpunar, C., J. B. Lambert, and J. E. Buikstra

1978 Analysis of excavated bone by atomic absorption. *American Journal of Physical Anthropology* 48:199–202.

Taylor, W. W.
1957 *The identification of non-artifactual archaeological materials.* Washington, D.C.: National Academy of Science—National Research Council Publication Number 565.

Thomas, D. H.
1971 On distinguishing natural from cultural bone in archeological sites. *American Antiquity 36*(3):366–371.

Thurber, D. L., J. L. Kulp, E. Hodges, P. W. Gast, and J. M. Wampler
1958 Common strontium content of the human skeleton. *Science 128:256–257.*

Toots, H., and M. R. Voorhies
1965 Strontium in fossil bones and the reconstruction of food chains. *Science 149:854–855.*

Towle, M. A.
1961 *The ethnobotany of pre-Columbian Peru.* Chicago: Aldine.

Trotter, M. and G. C. Gleser
1958 A re-evaluation of estimation of stature based on measurements of stature taken during life and of long bones after death. *American Journal of Physical Anthropology 16:79–124.*

United Nations
1955 Age and sex patterns of mortality, ST/SOA, Series A., *Population* (22).

United States Department of Agriculture
1953 Consumption of food in the United States, 1909–1952. USDA, Washington, D.C.

Vogel, J. C. and N. J. van der Merwe
1977 Isotopic evidence for early maize cultivation in New York state. *American Antiquity 42*(2):238–242.

Vogt, E. Z.
1974 *Aerial photography in anthropological field research.* Cambridge, Massachusetts: Harvard Univ. Press.

Voigt, E. A.
1975 Studies of marine mollusca from archaeological sites: Dietary preferences, environmental reconstruction and ethnological parallels. In *Archaeozoological Studies,* edited by A. T. Clason. Amsterdam: North Holland Press.

Vollweiler, L. G.
1978 Hunters, scapuli, and caribou. *The Florida Journal of Anthropology 3*(1):5–25.

Volman, T. P.
1978 Early archeological evidence for shellfish collection. *Science 201*(4359):911–913.

von den Driesch, A.
1976 A guide to the measurement of animal bones from archaeological sites. *Peabody Museum Bulletin* No. 1, Harvard University.

Von Endt, D. W.
1977 Amino-acid analysis of the contents of a vial excavated at Axum, Ethiopia. *Journal of Archaeological Science 4*(4):367–376.

Wagley, C.
1969 Cultural influences on population: A comparison of two Tupi tribes. In *Environment and cultural behavior,* edited by A. P. Vayda. New York: American Museum Sourcebooks in Anthropology, Natural History Press.

Watson, P. J.
1974 *Archeology of the Mammoth Cave Area.* New York: Academic Press.

Watson, P. J. and R. A. Yarnell
1966 Archaeological and Paleoethnobotanical investigations in Salts Cave, Mammoth Cave National Park, Kentucky. *American Antiquity 31*(6):842–849.

Watt, B. K., and A. L. Merrill
1963 *Composition of foods*. Agricultural Handbook No. 8, United States Department of Agriculture.

Waugh, F. W.
1973 *Iroquois foods and food preparation*. Department of Mines, Geological Survey Memoir 86, Facsimile Edition, Ottawa.

Weinmann, J. P., and H. Sicher
1947 *Bone and bones: Fundamentals of bone biology*. St. Louis: C.V. Mosby Co.

Weiss, K. M.
1973 Demographic models for anthropology. *Memoirs of the Society for American Archaeology* No. 27.

Wessen, G., F. Ruddy, C. Gustafson, and H. Irwin
1977 Characterization of archaeological bone by neutron activation analysis. *Archaeometry* 19:200–205.

Wheat, J. B.
1972 The Olsen-Chubbuck site: A Paleo-Indian bison kill. Memoirs of the *Society for American Archaeology* No. 26.

White, T. E.
1953a A method of calculating the dietary percentages of various food animals utilized by aboriginal peoples. *American Antiquity* 18(4):396–398.
1953b Observations of the butchering technique of some aboriginal peoples. *American Antiquity* 19(2):160–164.

Widdowson, E. R., and R. A. McCance
1960 *The composition of foods*, Medical Research Council Special Report Series No. 297. London: H.M. Stationery Office.

Wilke, P. J., and H. J. Hall
1975 Analysis of ancient feces: A discussion and annotated bibliography. *Archaeological Research Facility*. Mimeograph, Department of Anthropology, University of California, Berkeley.

Wilkinson, P. F.
1975 The relevance musk ox exploitation to the study of prehistoric animal economies. In *Paleoeconomy*, edited by E. S. Higgs. Cambridge, GB: University Press.

Williams, R. S. Jr., and W. D. Carter
1976 *ERTS-1 A new window on our planet*. Washington: U.S. Government Printing Office.

Wilmsen, E. N.
1978 Seasonal effects of dietary intake on Kalahari San. *Federation Proceedings* 37(1):65–72.

Wilson, R. H. L., and N. L. Wilson
1969 Obesity and respiratory stress. *Journal of American Diet Association* 55:465.

Woolley, D. W.
1963 *Metabolic inhibitors*. New York: Academic Press.

World Health Organization
Technical Report Series nos. 301, 362, 452, United Nations, New York.

Yablonskii, M. F.
1971 Use of differences in bone mineral content for identification of corpses. *Sbornik Nauchnykh Trudov Vitebskogo Gosudarstvennogo meditsinskogo Instituta* 14:368–374.
1973 Identificational significance of major and trace elements of human long tubular bones. *Sudebno-Meditsinskaya Ekspertiza* 16:16–18.

Zevallos, M. C., W. G. Galinat, D. W. Lathrap, E. R. Levy, J. G. Marcos, and K. M. Klumpp
  1977   The San Pablo corn kernel and its friends. *Science* 196(4288):385–389.
Ziegler, A. C.
  1973   Inference from prehistoric faunal remains. *Addison-Wesley Module in Anthropology* No. 43, Reading, Massachusetts.

Subject Index

Thomas F. King, Patricia Parker Hickman, and Gary Berg. **Anthropology in Historic Preservation: Caring for Culture's Clutter**

Richard E. Blanton. **Monte Albán: Settlement Patterns at the Ancient Zapotec Capital**

R. E. Taylor and Clement W. Meighan. **Chronologies in New World Archaeology**

Bruce D. Smith. **Prehistoric Patterns of Human Behavior: A Case Study in the Mississippi Valley**

Barbara L. Stark and Barbara Voorhies (Eds.). **Prehistoric Coastal Adaptations: The Economy and Ecology of Maritime Middle America**

Charles L. Redman, Mary Jane Berman, Edward V. Curtin, William T. Langhorne, Nina M. Versaggi, and Jeffery C. Wanser (Eds.). **Social Archeology: Beyond Subsistence and Dating**

Bruce D. Smith (Ed.). **Mississippian Settlement Patterns**

Lewis R. Binford. **Nunamiut Ethnoarchaeology**

J. Barto Arnold III and Robert Weddle. **The Nautical Archeology of Padre Island: The Spanish Shipwrecks of 1554**

Sarunas Milisauskas. **European Prehistory**

Brian Hayden (Ed.). **Lithic Use-Wear Analysis**

William T. Sanders, Jeffrey R. Parsons, and Robert S. Santley. **The Basin of Mexico: Ecological Processes in the Evolution of a Civilization**

David L. Clarke. **Analytical Archaeologist: Collected Papers of David L. Clarke. Edited and Introduced by His Colleagues**

Arthur E. Spiess. **Reindeer and Caribou Hunters: An Archaeological Study**

Elizabeth S. Wing and Antoinette B. Brown. **Paleonutrition: Method and Theory in Prehistoric Foodways.**

in preparation

John W. Rick. **Prehistoric Hunters of the High Andes**

Timothy K. Earle and Andrew L. Christenson (Eds.). **Modeling Change in Prehistoric Economics**